COPING WITH ALOPECIA

DR NIGEL HUNT obtained his BSc at Hatfield and PhD at [...] currently a Senior Lecturer [...] ham Trent University, [...] traumatic stress. He has written two books (a third one, on the treatment of war trauma, is forthcoming), and numerous articles in academic journals and elsewhere. Along with Dr Sue McHale, he is currently carrying out research examining the psychological impact of alopecia.

DR SUE McHALE obtained her BSc and PhD in Psychology at the University of Plymouth. She is currently a Senior Lecturer in Psychology at Sheffield Hallam University. She has a particular interest in the relationship between stress, illness and coping.

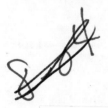

Overcoming Common Problems Series

Selected titles
A full list of titles is available from Sheldon Press,
1 Marylebone Road, London NW1 4DU, and on our website at
www.sheldonpress.co.uk

Overcoming Common Problems Series

Overcoming Common Problems Series

Overcoming Common Problems

Coping with Alopecia

Dr Nigel Hunt and Dr Sue McHale

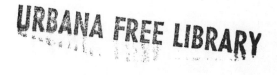

sheldon **PRESS**

First published in Great Britain in 2004 by
Sheldon Press
1 Marylebone Road
London NW1 4DU

© Dr Nigel Hunt and Dr Sue McHale 2004

British Library Cataloguing-in-Publication Data

A catalogue record for this book is available from the British Library

ISBN 0–85969–910–2

1 3 5 7 9 10 8 6 4 2

Typeset by Deltatype Limited, Birkenhead, Merseyside
Printed in Great Britain by Biddles Ltd
www.biddles.co.uk

Contents

1

Introduction

What is alopecia?

Greek: alopecia – a disease in which the hair falls out

Alopecia is a dermatological disorder whereby people lose some or all of the hair on their head and sometimes on their body as well. It is a chronic inflammatory disease that affects the hair follicles. It is neither life-threatening nor painful, though there can be irritation of the skin, particularly when undergoing treatment, and there can be physical problems associated with the loss of eyebrows and eyelashes. Unfortunately, it can be extremely psychologically damaging, causing intense emotional suffering and damage to relationships. One survey by Hairline International found that 40 per cent of women with alopecia had experienced problems in their marriages or long-term relationships. Many of these partnerships had broken up. On top of this, 63 per cent of those questioned said that they had also experienced career-related problems.

Most of us do not think about alopecia – until we get it ourselves or someone close to us gets it. The misery it causes goes unappreciated, and even medical professionals often ignore the impact it has on people's lives by treating it just like any other medical condition – which it is not. It can impact so severely on self-esteem that one's sense of self or identity is broken.

Alopecia is more common than many people think. We often don't notice people who have the disorder because they may cover up their hair loss by changing their hairstyle (perhaps shaving their head or brushing hair over the bald patch), or by wearing a wig. And it is very difficult to ascertain the number of people with the problem because many do not go to their GP, or tell others. Estimates vary from 0.1 per cent to 1 per cent of the population having alopecia at any given time, with a lifetime risk estimated at 1.7 per cent. It accounts for about 2 per cent of new dermatology outpatient attendances.

It can affect anyone, irrespective of sex, race (except for

Australian Aborigines), age, or socio-economic status – though there has been relatively little research carried out to assess the type, frequency or impact of alopecia on different ethnic and cultural groups, whether in the UK or elsewhere. For many, hair does not just have a significance relating to perceived attractiveness and identity – it may also have a cultural or religious significance. There does seem to be a family link, as one-fifth of people who have alopecia have a family history of the disease. With regard to age, 60 per cent of patients present with alopecia for the first time before they are 20.

There is also an association between alopecia and autoimmune diseases, which suggests the possibility that alopecia is itself an autoimmune disease. (This will be discussed in detail in Chapter 3.)

How does alopecia differ from ordinary baldness?

We need to distinguish between alopecia and ordinary baldness. This book is not mainly concerned with the latter, though some of the psychological issues are relevant – both for men and women. Many men lose their hair naturally over a number of years, usually between the ages of 20 and 60. There are 'treatments' on the market for male-pattern baldness, but it is a perfectly natural phenomenon that most men come to terms with relatively easily. In contrast, alopecia is a disorder that affects anyone – men, women and children – and can have very serious effects on someone's life, striking quickly and without obvious cause.

What happens when someone gets alopecia?

For a minority, particularly those undergoing chemotherapy, the course of alopecia is predictable. Hair is likely to fall out during the treatment, and is likely to grow back again when this is stopped. However, for most people there is no prior warning that they are going to get alopecia, and often the first clue is finding more hairs than usual when washing your hair. It is something people do not worry about too much to begin with – it is only when the hair starts to fall out in chunks that it becomes a problem.

In some people, it is not only the hair that is affected, but also fingernails. This may involve pinprick indentations on the surface of the nail, or the nails themselves can become distorted.

There is some evidence of a link between alopecia and other disorders such as eczema, allergies and asthma.

But remember, the one thing we *do* know about alopecia is that it's not contagious!

Is it permanent?

For some people alopecia is a permanent disfigurement, for others it is temporary, perhaps occurring after an illness, an injury, or a stressful event. You might lose your hair quite suddenly, and then almost as suddenly it can start growing back again – weeks, months or even years later. We cannot predict when hair will grow back or in what form – sometimes it will grow back normally, sometimes it grows back much thinner and more wispy. We do not know for sure that hair will grow back, although it is far more likely to regrow if the hair loss is limited to patches on the scalp. When all the body hair falls out, there is a much lower chance of regrowth.

It is thought that somewhere between 50 per cent and 80 per cent of people with alopecia have hair regrowth within one year. However, the problem is that the disorder may recur, perhaps several times during a person's lifetime.

As we have already said, alopecia can affect you in different ways. Some people lose small patches of hair, others lose all their head hair, and some lose all their body hair too.

If you have less severe hair loss you are more likely to experience full hair regrowth, possibly in weeks or months; but if you have more severe hair loss, the hair may reappear but only as a light wispy covering. For many, particularly those with the most severe hair loss, the hair never grows back. For those with repeated occurrences of alopecia, it may be in the same places, but it can also be in different places – sometimes more serious, sometimes less serious.

The important thing to remember, though, is that there is no loss of hair follicles with alopecia, so there will always be the *possibility* of hair regrowth, even with the most severe cases. But it is important not to rely on regrowth – there is also the chance that you may have to learn to live with alopecia.

3

Can alopecia be treated?

There is a range of medical treatments available on the market, but the evidence for their effectiveness is rather weak. The treatments can be painful; also, they may work for some people and not for others. They can work temporarily or permanently. Research into the effectiveness of treatments for alopecia is difficult to carry out because so many people (particularly with the more mild forms of the disease) spontaneously recover that it is difficult to be sure, without randomized controlled trials, whether it is the treatment that has helped or whether someone's hair would have grown back anyway. A randomized control study would involve taking a group of people with alopecia and randomly allocating them either to a treatment or a control group. Any difference in remission rates between the two groups would indicate the success of the treatment.

A further problem is that experimental trials have often focused on the more severe forms of alopecia, where spontaneous remission is rare. Yet treatments that do not work with this group may still have value with the milder forms of alopecia. Furthermore, there is evidence that some treatments work while the treatment is ongoing, but once treatment stops the hair falls out again.

What causes alopecia?

The simple answer is that we do not know for sure, although there are a number of factors associated with the onset of alopecia. Possible causes include a change in the immunological system, a genetic link, and psychological causes – and there is evidence for all three. (This will be explored in more detail in Chapter 3.) We do know that around 20 per cent of people with alopecia know of someone else in their family who also has the disorder – sometimes identical twins both get alopecia. In a genetically prone individual there may be a range of factors that could trigger the disorder, although the most likely reasons involve a combination of genetic and environmental factors.

What is the relationship between alopecia and illness?

As we have already mentioned, alopecia is associated with a number of diseases and problems, both physical and psychological. It can be a cause of another disorder, a consequence of the other disorder, or a concomitant disorder.

For example, people with skin-related problems (not only alopecia, but also acne, eczema and psoriasis) tend to have a higher rate of psychiatric disorders than the general population, and people with alopecia experience more neurotic depression than people without alopecia. They also experience more generalized anxiety, depression and phobic states. However, it is often very difficult to establish whether the alopecia is a *cause* or a *consequence* of these psychological disorders. It does seem likely, though, that there is some kind of genetic predisposition towards both psychiatric disorders and alopecia. (We will explore this in more detail later in the book.)

What we don't know

By now it will have become clear that there is a lot we don't know about alopecia and its causes. The reasons for the disorder obviously vary from person to person – it could have a psychological cause, it could be the result of a physical trauma such as an injury to the head, or it could be genetic. Also, as mentioned above, there are a lot of treatments available, but we cannot predict with any certainty who will respond to them, and who will not.

If you, or someone close to you has alopecia, no doubt this all sounds very pessimistic, but it is best from the outset to be as honest as we can about the problem. Alopecia can be a serious disfigurement disorder, one that causes a great deal of distress to the sufferer. We do not have a guaranteed cure, but there are certainly ways in which we can make life easier for the person with alopecia. There is advice that can, if used well, reduce the distress and suffering.

Of course, for those with more serious forms of alopecia, where eyebrows and eyelashes fall out, there are added issues of psychological and physical discomfort. The loss of eyebrows and eyelashes fundamentally changes the face of the individual, and can also create practical problems. For example, water gets in the eyes (because brows and lashes provide protection, like guttering on a house); and eyes become sore because without lashes the eyelid turns in on itself and the cornea can become scratched.

So while we still do not know enough about alopecia to be able to effectively treat it, we do know enough about people to provide appropriate support and guidance, to help cope with the problems that arise as a result of alopecia – a main aim of this book.

Wigs

People with alopecia, particularly women, commonly use wigs. Wigs are, for many, the most effective means of coping with the social world. Women's wigs tend to look more natural than men's – perhaps because more women use wigs so there is a bigger market, perhaps because appearance is more important for women than for men – so women demand higher standards. In the UK, wigs can be obtained via the NHS. (The subject of wigs is explored in more detail later in the book.)

Types of alopecia

Alopecia is classified according to its severity – in other words, the extent to which someone's hair is lost. There are many different types of alopecia, the most frequent of which is alopecia areata.

Alopecia areata

This is where you lose some, but not all, of your head hair. This usually occurs in patches, on any part of the head. It often begins with a single round patch of baldness, which can quickly spread. It can occur on other parts of the body, but it is more frequent and more noticeable on the scalp. It may be a single patch of hair loss, perhaps just a centimetre or two in diameter. It is more likely to occur at the back of the head than at the front for males, and more often towards the front for females. Some people experience repeated alopecia areata in the same area; some have it in different areas. Men might have alopecia in the beard. If you have alopecia areata you can often cover up the bald patch on your head with the rest of the hair. The prognosis for this type of alopecia is generally good – you are likely to experience hair regrowth, where the hair grows back as normal, though you may lose it again in the future. But this is not necessarily the case: for some, the hair grows back as a fluffy patch that does not match the rest of the hair, and for others it does not grow back at all. Overall, though, it is the least serious form of alopecia.

About 65 per cent of people with alopecia areata only experience one or two patches of hair loss, which often regrows spontaneously after a few weeks or months. Alopecia areata is unpredictable – some people only have a single bout of it, others experience it repeatedly. Sometimes the new hair growth is very fine and unpigmented; on other occasions it grows back normally. Regrowth can occur in one area, at the same time as another bald patch is appearing elsewhere.

Alopecia totalis

This occurs when you lose all your head hair, but not your body hair – and (usually) not eyelashes and eyebrows. The prognosis is not as good as for alopecia areata, although many people do experience at least some regrowth. This regrowth may occur in patches, and it may only be fine wispy hair. Figures vary, but the British Association of Dermatologists estimates that 14–25 per cent of people with alopecia have alopecia totalis.

Alopecia universalis (or alopecia disseminata)

This is where you lose all your head and body hair, including your eyelashes and eyebrows, along with underarm and genital hair. This is the most severe form of alopecia, but it is also the rarest. The prognosis for someone with alopecia universalis is not very good, for few will achieve total regrowth of hair. It is estimated that less than 10 per cent of people with alopecia universalis will experience full recovery.

It is not clear exactly how many people with alopecia areata will go on to develop totalis or universalis – estimates vary from 7 per cent to 30 per cent.

Alopecia androgenetica

This is commonly known as ordinary baldness, or male-pattern baldness. As mentioned earlier, this is not the focus of this book as hair loss in the male is normal, and generally does not cause intense distress. However, there *are* occasions when it can become a problem – both for men and for women. In these cases this book may be of some help.

Although ordinary baldness is more common in men, it also occurs in some women. It often appears as thinning hair across most or all of the head. It often occurs after the menopause, but it can also happen in younger women who are genetically predisposed to the condition. It can be triggered by eating disorders and by the progesterone present in some contraceptive pills. This form of alopecia can be just as serious a problem for women as the other forms of alopecia.

Other forms of alopecia and hair loss

There are other forms of alopecia, such as alopecia medicamentosa, where hair loss is caused by some medical treatment (such as chemotherapy), or alopecia congenitalis, where a child is born with no hair.

Alopecia diffusa is where the individual loses some hair across a large part of their scalp or body, and this can be difficult to distinguish from other forms of hair loss. The real difference is that alopecia diffusa tends to be more serious; it can be a progressive hair loss.

Another type of the disorder, alopecia barbae, is specific to men and affects only the beard.

Telogen effluvium is a human moulting condition that occurs after the body has experienced a severe trauma. It can occur after a high fever, childbirth, or extreme shock.

Trichotillomania is the term given to the condition whereby people have an obsessive compulsive disorder that leads them to pull out their own hair.

Counselling

If you have alopecia you can become profoundly upset and disturbed by the hair loss, so it is important that you can discuss your disorder, and its likely course, with a specialist. If you have alopecia you need to know the truth about the illness, and be aware that many medical treatments have limited effectiveness, and that there may be relapse after treatment. On the other hand, as already noted, hair regrowth occurs spontaneously for many.

The problems experienced, particularly by women and by children, must be taken into account in any counselling offered. Children may experience problems at school, such as bullying and name-calling, or being ostracized. Women may have difficulties because their hair is central to their appearance. A bald-headed man is fairly normal; a bald-headed woman is not – at least, not in Western society.

For some, support groups such as Hairline International and Changing Faces, or the website www.keratin.com, are useful (see Further Information at the back of this book). They provide opportunities to discuss alopecia with fellow sufferers, and to learn from others how they adapt to and cope with their hair loss.

Alopecia is a form of disfigurement, and it can lead to massive changes in the ways you perceive yourself personally and socially, at home, at school and at work. Those who do not suffer from alopecia generally have little understanding of the impact it can have on someone. People have been known to lose their jobs because of their appearance. One of the purposes of this book is to try and increase awareness and understanding of the problem. Only by discussing the subject in some detail, exploring what it means to have alopecia, can we help those who suffer with the condition. The rest of the book will hopefully go some way towards this enlightenment.

Jake

Jake had a head of dark thick hair of which he was particularly proud. In August, Jake had become a father. In November, his best friend died in a car crash. This was a devastating experience, and was to have a permanent impact on his life. Within weeks he noticed that chunks of his hair started to fall out in the bath and in the shower. At first he thought little of it, but when he realized that there were gaps appearing on his scalp he went to see his GP. Jake knew nothing of alopecia.

His GP immediately said that Jake had alopecia, and recommended that he should see a dermatologist, a skin specialist. Jake assumed that the dermatologist would be able to determine exactly what was wrong and would provide a cure. By this time Jake was starting to have difficulties going out in public. There were more bare patches than hair on his scalp, and when he went out he thought everyone was looking at him and laughing.

The dermatologist prescribed minoxidil, a steroid treatment. The cream had to be rubbed into the scalp at regular intervals. Jake's hair was still falling out, along with his eyebrows and eyelashes. His whole appearance changed, and his partner, the mother of his baby, stopped looking him in the eye. In fact, she never looked him in the eye again.

Within six months of the death of his friend, Jake had alopecia universalis – total hair loss. There remained not a single hair on his whole body. He felt a freak, and dared not expose his head in public. He felt he couldn't shower in public sports halls. The only person who did not seem to notice was his son.

2
Hair

What is hair?

To understand alopecia we need first to learn about hair. What is hair? Why do we have it? How does it grow? Why does it fall out?

Skin is the second largest organ in the body, and has a range of functions, including: supporting the body, protecting internal organs, temperature control, excretion (e.g. sweat), vitamin formation, sensation and immunological defence.

While there are huge variations, on average we have five million hairs on our body, and between 100,000 and 150,000 of these are on our scalp. This varies quite substantially according to your hair colour. Blond people tend to have more hairs, redheads fewer. Nearly every part of our bodies are covered with hair apart from the palms of our hands, the soles of our feet, lips, and parts of our genitalia.

Why do we have hair?

The main purpose of hair is temperature control. Mammals need a fairly stable body temperature, and the hair – or fur – on mammals is important in keeping warm. Hair has some flexibility depending on the outside temperature. For example, goose bumps occur when a muscle attached to the hair follicle contracts, causing the hair to stand on end. In animals that have fur, this causes warm air to be trapped between the hairs that form a layer to keep the animal warm. Other animals, e.g. otters, use hair to trap a layer of air around their bodies for buoyancy.

Hair also has a role in sexual maturity and health. There are secondary sex characteristics relating to hair (e.g. beard), and in many animals the quality of hair is a determination of health and vitality; and hence attractiveness to the opposite sex. Hair can also act as camouflage, protection against ultraviolet light, or in cuts and bruises. Eyelashes and eyebrows protect the eyes, and nasal hair protects the lungs from invasive particles.

The main role of hair for humans today, though, is cosmetic. We have other means of controlling temperature (e.g. fire, clothes), but we still use hair to make ourselves attractive (or so we like to think!). Hairdressers can earn a lot of money telling people they need to have elaborate and expensive hairstyles; and there are many products available to remove unwanted hair. The beauty industry is worth billions (choose your currency) each year. Hundreds of shampoos, conditioners, hair products of all kinds are available, and we are bombarded with the benefits of this form of hair gel or that kind of hair spray. People are encouraged to change their hair colour using 'natural' dyes. There are products to 'strengthen hair', or to give it 'lustre'. Whether or not any of these products have actual physical benefits is largely irrelevant. The point is that hair is seen as a key part of physical attractiveness, and the cosmetic industry caters for that.

What is hair made of?

Hair is made of a protein called keratin. Keratin is also found in our nails (which may explain why many people with alopecia also have problems with their fingernails).

Hair has three layers:

1 *Cuticle*: The outer layer that is transparent and protects the inner layers.
2 *Cortex*: The middle layer, the strongest part of the hair.
3 *Medulla*: The inner layer, composed of large cells that may appear hollow.

The hair follicle

Hairs grow from hair follicles, which are sac-like structures in the skin that surround the root of the hair; sebaceous glands at the hair root secrete sebum oil, which protects hair, keeping it in good condition.

Papillae, at the base of the hair follicle, are fed by blood vessels. Papillae are sensitive to hormones and chemicals that affect hair growth, either helping it grow – or stopping it. Pigmented cells called melanocytes, which contain melanin, determine hair colour, and it is the amount of melanin that determines this colour. There are two types of melanin, eumelanin, which turns the hair from brown to black, and pheomelanin, which colours hair from blond to red.

Our first hair

Our hair starts growing before we are born, although we still do not know what triggers this, or why. The first hair we have is called lanugo (which is Latin for fine wool). This is usually shed around the time of birth, to be replaced with our more familiar hair (though lanugo may return after alopecia). The pattern of hair, the whorls, varies between people, and is related to the formation of hair follicles as the skin is stretched over the growing foetus.

The hair cycle

There are three phases to the hair cycle:

1 *The anagen phase*: This is when the hair is actively growing, and is the longest phase of the cycle, lasting anything from two to ten years. Up to 90 per cent of hair cells are in this phase at any one time.
2 *The catagen phase*: This is when the hair is resting.
3 *The telogen phase*: This is when the hair is being shed, and lasts between one and three months. A hair must be shed in order to prepare for the next anagen or growing phase.

The cycle of any particular hair cell is independent of the cycle of the hair cells surrounding it, so the loss of a single hair is generally not perceptible because many cells around will be in the anagen or growing phase.

People lose many hairs every day of their lives – somewhere between 40 and 120 hairs on average just from the scalp. If we lost 100 hairs a day and they were not replaced, we would lose all our hair in less than three years. Fortunately (for most people), the hair is replaced. Around 90 per cent of head hair is growing, at approximately 1 centimetre a month, but the rate varies according to individual differences, emotional factors, nutrition, hormones, age (hair grows more slowly in older people) and the site of the follicle. It also varies according to the season, with hair growing more quickly in summer than in winter. Each hair grows for between two and ten years. When the growth phase ends, the hair follicle has a few months of rest and the hair is lost. Only about 10 per cent of hair is in the resting phase. After this, there is another growth phase.

Hair loss

A hair cell in the telogen phase will lose the hair for a number of reasons, though it is normally through activities such as combing/ brushing and washing. As we mentioned earlier, hair loss can occur because of certain medical treatments (e.g. radiotherapy or chemo- therapy), or as a result of a physical trauma (e.g. burns). There are also the psychological states that lead to loss – for instance, conditions such as trichotillomania (repetitive hair pulling). In other people, excessive hair loss may occur because of particular hairstyles, such as ones where the hair is pulled tightly away from the scalp, such as in ponytails or braids.

Ordinary male baldness

A number of hormones impact on the way hair growth occurs. Dihydrotestosterone (DHT), which is made from testosterone, acts on hair follicles, causing growth to slow and eventually stop. It works only on particular hair follicles that have the genetic predisposition to be shut down. These are usually on the top of our heads, and result in male-pattern balding.

The issues surrounding the personal and social consequences of hair loss, and coping and adapting to such loss, which are discussed in the second half of the book, will have relevance to some people who have ordinary baldness.

3
Causes of alopecia

Problems in identifying the causes of alopecia

It is only in recent years that scientists have carried out much research into the causes of alopecia, and there is still a lot of disagreement among researchers as to why people develop this condition. A number of explanations have been put forward, and there is probably some truth in many of them. There often appears to be a psychological cause in alopecia – some sufferers have some sort of shock, a stressful or traumatic incident, that makes their hair fall out. Some recent research suggests that sufferers have a genetic predisposition, but the favoured theory is that people with alopecia have a dysfunctional immune system.

This chapter will try to answer this difficult question with regard to causes. We do need to understand something about the cause of a disorder in order to find the best ways of treating it. If you don't have a biological training or scientific background, you might find some of the terms used somewhat daunting, but persevere! In order to deal successfully with your alopecia you need to try to understand it. There is a Glossary at the back of the book that helps to explain many of these terms.

Problems with undertaking research into alopecia

There are numerous problems that arise when scientists try to understand why people get alopecia. These include:

- The *range* of disorders that people experience – alopecia areata, alopecia totalis and alopecia universalis. It is still not clear whether these are all variations of the same disorder or whether they are totally separate disorders, possibly with different causes. (Of course, alopecia also occurs as a consequence of chemotherapy – of which more later.)
- The difficulty in establishing exactly who has alopecia. Many cases go unrecognized by the medical community because people

do not report the problem, or their condition is not recorded – and little research has been carried out to find out who has alopecia. There are no studies that have identified the number of alopecia cases in the population to provide appropriate samples for research.

- The difficulty of isolating potential causes. Is alopecia caused by stress? Is it an immunological disorder? The picture is very complicated, and we need to make further technological advances before we can examine and understand immunological and genetic issues.

Early ideas relating to the causes of alopecia

Since the first use of the term 'alopecia' by Sauvages in his *Nosologica Medica*, written in 1760, there have been a variety of causes suggested. During the nineteenth century there were two main schools of thought on this. The first was that it was caused by a parasitic infection, an idea first put forward by Gruby in 1843. The second theory came in 1858, when Von Barensrung suggested that alopecia might be caused by a nervous disorder – or what we would now call stress. The idea of a parasitic infection was proposed because of the way in which many types of alopecia appear to spread outwards from a single site; and also because there were observed outbreaks in schools and orphanages, which seemed to show that alopecia is 'catching'. Unfortunately, despite many attempts to isolate the 'infection', and to transfer alopecia via inoculation, there has been no success in supporting the parasitic hypothesis, and doctors long ago rejected it.

The second school of thought – that alopecia is a nervous or stress-related disorder – became very popular towards the end of the nineteenth century. It was referred to as the 'neuropathic hypothesis', or the 'trophoneurotic hypothesis'. Support for this hypothesis came by way of observed links between emotional stress and hair loss. It was thought that emotional distress caused damage to the hair follicles via damage to the nervous system. In 1886 Joseph attempted to prove this by showing that alopecia could be brought about by cutting the nerves in the necks of cats. The cats then experienced hair loss. Unfortunately, as is the case so often in

16

science, conditions were not fully controlled and it later became clear that the hair loss was a result of the cats scratching themselves! Similar ideas tried to associate alopecia with tooth decay and with eyestrain – they too were not successful!

Just before the First World War, Sabouraud put forward the theory that alopecia was associated with disorders of the endocrine glands, particularly the thyroid. This was a very popular hypothesis, and led to a lot of research on the topic. In fact, it does seem that there is a link between thyroid problems and hair loss.

Alopecia has also in the past been linked to diseases such as syphilis. People with syphilis may lose their hair, often in patches, in a similar way to people with alopecia areata. Syphilis can also affect the fingernails – something else associated with alopecia. No doubt this caused a great deal of mental distress to people in the days before antibiotics could control syphilis. Indeed, people with alopecia were often ostracized because others thought they had syphilis. It should be made clear that there is *not* a link between the two disorders!

Another hypothesis proposed in the early twentieth century was that alopecia developed because of the introduction of some poison that induced hair loss. This was supported by research showing that the injection of rat poison could lead to alopecia. This is another idea that has now been abandoned.

Modern ideas about the causes of alopecia

As already noted, we are still a long way from fully understanding the causes of alopecia, but we have a number of ideas that are worth exploring. These include psychological causes such as chronic stress or sudden traumatic stress, and a range of physical causes such as physical injury, skin damage, a genetic predisposition, a viral or bacterial infection, hormonal changes, allergies, environmental chemicals and seasonal changes. The main hypothesis, though, is that alopecia is an autoimmune disorder.

Alopecia as an autoimmune disorder

Many dermatologists now believe that alopecia is an autoimmune disorder. An autoimmune disease is one where the person's own immune system mistakes part of his or her body tissue for an invading foreign organism, and so attacks it, attempting to destroy it. There is increasing evidence for this hypothesis.

Psychoneuroimmunology
The science of psychoneuroimmunology is exciting for both psychologists and medical practitioners. It is the science (*logy*) of the mind (*psycho*), the brain and nervous system (*neuro*) and the immune system (*immuno*), and how they interact. If psychological factors do play a role in autoimmune disorders such as arthritis, asthma and alopecia, then they may help regulate the immune system, and so psychological interventions should be able to help bring about a cure (see Chapter 8 for psychological aids to recovery).

The immune system
The immune system is very complicated. We do not need a detailed account of it here, but it is useful to know something about it because it is thought to be associated very closely with alopecia. (There is a book cited in Further Information for those who are interested in knowing more about this.)

The main cells of the immune system are known as leucocytes or white blood cells. These are the 'guards' of the body. They 'patrol' the blood supply by looking for 'invaders', such as infection or cell damage (perhaps caused by a cut or a bruise). Once they discover such an invasion, extra cells are despatched from the lymph nodes to counter the invader and destroy it.

There are several types of white blood cell, which have different roles in the system. We are particularly interested in lymphocytes, of which there are various types, including B cells, NK cells and T cells. B cells control infection; and NK (natural killer) cells destroy virus-infected and tumour cells. T cells can be further subdivided into: T helper cells, which enhance immune function by stimulating the replication of immune system cells and antibodies; cytotoxic T cells, which destroy parasites, virus- and tumour-infected cells; and T suppressor cells, which inhibit immune responses. As we shall see, T cells are implicated in alopecia.

It would be very convenient if we could talk about the immune system as being enhanced or suppressed, and that the former protects while the latter is caused by stress and leads to illness. Unfortunately, it is not that simple! The functioning of the immune system is both complex and constantly changing. Something that enhances one part might suppress another. The number and type of cells active in a healthy body varies between individuals and changes constantly within individuals, so the system is very difficult to understand.

Stress is linked to immune function. Exactly how this works is not yet known, but research has shown some interesting links. One consistent finding is that chronic stress is linked to a decrease in certain types of immune cells, particularly NK cells and T cells. Short-term stressors make the immune system more effective – for example, the body fights infection immediately after a traumatic injury. But stress over a longer period of time results in a *decrease* in the effectiveness of the system. In other words, this suggests that in the short term the body can cope with stress, but if it *persists*, over time physical problems may arise.

Alopecia and the immune system
Originally, the idea that alopecia is an immune disorder came from observations that if a person is undergoing some form of immuno-suppressive therapy, then they often get alopecia. Also, immune cells are commonly observed around hair follicles that are not working; and alopecia is found in conjunction with other autoimmune diseases.

So the idea that alopecia is an immune disorder is currently very popular among researchers, but how this works in detail is not known and a lot of the ideas are still only hypotheses.

How does the immune system cause alopecia?
We cannot be certain of the exact relationship between alopecia and immune function, but there are three possibilities:

1 *Autoimmunity leads to alopecia.*
   This means that the activity of the immune system leads to alopecia, and that for some reason immune cells treat the hair follicle as alien, and attack it – causing hair to fall out.
2 *Alopecia leads to immune dysfunction.*
   This is the least likely hypothesis. In this scenario, the hair falls out and this leads to immune activity. In other words, the loss of the hair cells results in antigens being produced, which leads to immune activity around the affected area.

3 *The third possibility.*

It could be that hair loss and immune dysfunction are not linked. Perhaps a third factor, such as infection, is causing alopecia.

The presence of immune cells around the alopecia-affected area is not understood. We do not know why they are there.

Even if alopecia *is* an autoimmune disorder, that does not mean that the effects will be permanent. A shock might tip the balance back into proper function (and hair growth). On the other hand, once an autoimmune disease is initiated it can be self-perpetuating. If the immune system destroys body tissue, then the resulting antigens (these are usually proteins and act as markers for the immune cells) are presented to immune system cells in the lymph nodes. This will then lead to further self-reactive cells destroying yet more tissue, which produces more antigens and so on.

Hair cells in the growth phase are attacked by the immune cells, which causes the cells to pass quickly through the resting phase and shed the hair fibre in the telogen phase. In the majority of people with alopecia this starts in a single small area and gradually spreads outwards, causing the characteristic circles of alopecia patches, though people with alopecia totalis or universalis may find that hair falls out uniformly – and this may indicate that they are in fact different disorders. If the hair cell tries to re-enter the growth phase, it sometimes produces a weak and distorted hair (the cell is described as being in a 'dystrophic anagen phase'). These hair cells can continue to move between the anagen and telogen phases, with the hair growing a little and then falling out. For some this may continue permanently, for others the hair cell eventually stays in the telogen phase, and stops growing altogether.

We do not know what causes these problems, and why the immune system starts to attack the hair. We still need to identify an autoantigen, something that triggers the immune attack. We do not know whether this antigen is a normal antigen that is exposed by an external trigger (e.g. stress), whether it is an abnormal follicular antigen, or whether there is some other immune system malfunction. Whatever the mechanism, the structure appears to protect against follicular damage. This is important if you have alopecia. It shows that the hair follicle, even after years of being attacked by the immune system, remains capable of regeneration.

Psychological factors

There is a lot of evidence to suggest that alopecia may be caused by stress – indeed, it is such an important subject that we have devoted the whole of the next chapter to it. We do not have definitive evidence for a causal link, but there is a great deal of work showing an association between stressful events and the onset of alopecia. However, not all researchers accept that stress can be a cause of alopecia, so we have yet another area of ongoing debate. Again, research in this area is difficult, particularly because of problems in establishing proper control groups for comparison.

The biggest problem when trying to determine the relationship between stress and alopecia is that alopecia itself can cause stress, so that complicates the picture. If you have alopecia and are feeling distressed, is it because you were under a lot of stress beforehand or does having alopecia cause the stress? The studies are all retrospective, in that they look back at a person's life, and ask them to report what happened, so it can be very difficult to determine whether a high level of stress is a cause or a consequence of alopecia – or both.

There is, though, a direct link between *perceived* stress and disease, and many studies have shown that perceived stress (i.e. if someone *feels* they are suffering from stress) relates to immune function and physical disorders. That is, the successful functioning of the immune system depends on how we perceive the stress in our environment, and we are of course all very different. Two people having the same experience – say, sitting an exam – may view it very differently. One person may be very confident, take the exam in their stride, and not get distressed. The other may lack confidence and become very distressed simply by the thought of the exam. It is the latter who is most likely to experience an immune disorder.

There is evidence that alopecia is linked not only to ordinary stressful events, but also to traumatic stress. There have been many reports that sudden highly stressful events, such as the death of a family member, or a war or rape experience, can lead to alopecia. In 1980 the American Psychiatric Association introduced the term 'post-traumatic stress disorder' (PTSD), meaning a disorder resulting from such traumatic events. The symptoms include re-experiencing the event in terms of traumatic memories, flashbacks or nightmares; avoidance of reminders of the event; emotional numbing; and physiological symptoms such as a heightened startle reflex or the inability to concentrate. Not everybody exposed to a traumatic event gets PTSD. On the other hand, we do know that some people are *somaticizers* – in other words, they do not get psychological symptoms, but instead subconsciously translate their feelings into a physical problem. There is a lot of evidence that at least a proportion of people with alopecia got it after a traumatic event.

As for ordinary stressful events, there are big differences in the ways people respond to traumatic events, though we do not fully understand the reasons why. It may be due to differences in biological make-up, personality, or favoured ways of coping, or perceived lack of support from family and friends.

PTSD introduces a complication into our understanding of alopecia because, just like alopecia, it can have a major impact on the way we view ourselves and the world. Just as alopecia is a disfigurement that can seriously disrupt the self, PTSD is a psychological injury that disrupts the self. The combination of the two can be incredibly damaging. While a traumatic event can lead to PTSD and alopecia, it is also the case that alopecia can *itself* be a traumatic event which leads to PTSD – doubling the problem.

There is a possibility that stress may lead to alopecia in people who already have a genetic predisposition for the disorder.

Attachment theory

Attachment theory was originally put forward after the war by John Bowlby to explain why some children behave badly and some behave well. 'Attachment' relates to how securely 'attached' a child is to their parent, and affects the degree of security that the child feels. Securely attached children will not be too distressed when their parents leave the room; insecurely attached children will cry and have tantrums. It has been shown that the attachment style in infancy can predict attachment style in later life, so secure attachment at a young age predicts stability through life. If there are problems with attachment when the child is young, this predicts later problems.

Attachment theory has been linked to coping with alopecia. We will look at coping in more detail in Chapter 8, but for now it is worth noting that the ways in which people cope with any sort of problem can predict the outcome of that problem. If you cope well, then you are likely to have a more favourable outcome than if you do not cope well. As attachment is linked to successful coping, then it is an important concept.

There is biological evidence relating to attachment and emotional expression that shows that rigid styles of emotion cause larger discrepancies between different levels of coping in insecurely attached individuals than in securely attached individuals. Attachment styles appear to be linked to maladaptive health behaviour and perceived symptoms. People who report more physical complaints, and those who are somaticizers, have more anxious attachment patterns. People with unexplained physical symptoms have higher insecure attachment and more psychiatric problems.

Alopecia and personality

There is a range of theories that examine personality and the way that it can affect our responses to events and illnesses. For example, there is strong evidence that specific personality traits are connected with certain diseases such as peptic ulcers, coronary heart diseases, hypertension and a variety of skin complaints. At one time researchers used terms like 'asthmatic personality' and 'ulcerous personality'. Fortunately, those terms are no longer in use (what is an 'alopecic personality'?), and research is more concerned with the interaction between traits and disease (psychosomatic medicine).

There may be a link between alopecia and neuroticism, with neurotic people more likely to experience alopecia. (Neuroticism, or 'negative aspect', is where a person is more likely to view events negatively.) One study showed that people with alopecia have high rates of depression, phobic-obsessive disorders and hysterical traits. Another study found that people with alopecia tended to have Type A personalities – that is, they are characterized by domination, aggressiveness, pathological competitivity, impulsiveness, impatience, the desire to achieve many goals in a short time, hyperactivity and explosiveness.

Italian researchers have explored another interesting area of study. They have focused on alexithymia, which is a disorder whereby people have problems in expressing emotions, and describing experiences and subjective feelings. One study found that 66 per cent of people with alopecia had alexithymia – an unusual finding considering that alexithymia is a relatively rare disorder.

The problems with personality research are that personality

researchers do not agree on how we should classify and measure personality, nor do the studies show consistent results. There is also the problem that personality affects the outcome of alopecia, and alopecia impacts on personality, so it is difficult to draw any firm conclusions from the research that has been carried out.

Genetic predisposition

As already indicated, there is a genetic predisposition to alopecia, with a greater incidence of alopecia among genetically related individuals. There is also evidence that particular genes are more common in people with alopecia than in the general population. This research is promising. It is only in the last few years that scientists have really begun to understand our genetic structure and the role that specific genes play in physical attributes and behaviour. If you are genetically predisposed to alopecia, this does not mean you will definitely suffer from it, or even that you are particularly *likely* to experience the disorder, but it does mean that if you are exposed to particular environmental variables then there may be a fair chance of you developing alopecia. It is very likely that this genetic predisposition is linked not to a single gene, but to a pattern of genes (i.e. it is what scientists call polygenetic).

Evidence for a genetic predisposition has been obtained from family studies. For instance, around 20 per cent of patients with alopecia report having other members of the family who have it. The figures vary. One study examined 348 severely affected patients and found that 16 per cent had a relative with alopecia. A child who has a parent with alopecia has a 6 per cent risk of developing the condition. If one identical twin gets alopecia, there is a high chance the other will as well.

Alopecia occurs in most ethnic groups, though one study showed that no cases of alopecia have been reported in Australian Aborigines of non-mixed race.

The disorder has been observed in many animals too – including dogs, cats, horses, cattle and other primates – and this information has been used to try to identify the role of specific genes. Most animal research has used rodents, and one of the main animals used is the Dundee Experimental Bald Rat (DEBR). The DEBR has been genetically developed to have hair loss. Understanding the role of alopecia-related genes in the rat may help researchers to identify the alopecia-related genes in humans. We may be able to do this because humans and rats share at least 80 per cent of genes.

There is the association between genes and the immune system. Certain proteins have the capacity to present a particular antigen, so the genes that are linked to these proteins may increase the follicular immune attack.

The pattern of genes varies according to whether the person has patchy alopecia areata or alopecia totalis, providing further evidence that the various kinds of alopecia are distinct disorders.

Research has suggested that the causes for alopecia are complex. In other words, we *all* have a threshold for susceptibility for alopecia. If genetic and environmental factors interact in a particular way, then we cross the threshold and develop alopecia. Put another way, in order to get alopecia, we must have a particular combination of genes, and particular environmental experiences. The genetic component can be split into those genes that provide the risk that someone will get alopecia, and those genes that are linked to the severity of the disorder. But before we can work out exactly what these gene combinations are, we must find a way of defining the *phenotype* of alopecia (how the disease is expressed), so we can carry out genetic studies using consistent criteria.

Carrying out this genetic work is a very difficult task, because – as we have said – not everyone with alopecia goes to see their doctor; others may not even realize they have the condition. Then there is the difficulty of establishing the role of environmental factors, and personality and temperament characteristics. By and large, as noted, alopecia is thought to be a polygenetic disease, with some genes responsible for susceptibility and others concerned with severity. The interaction between genetic and environmental factors, it seems, is what triggers the disease.

Genetic therapy is one area (still contentious) that might hold promise of a cure for alopecia. (This area is explored in Chapter 6.)

Other possible causes

Alopecia can be caused by injury to the scalp, and people who experience such injuries, and who are already susceptible to the condition, often experience new patches of hair loss in the surrounding areas. On the other hand, such an injury in an area already affected by alopecia can lead to hair *regrowth* – so it is no wonder that scientists are having such difficulty in establishing exactly what is going on! Injuries in an affected area can promote anagen follicle growth in the skin immediately surrounding the damaged site.

Viral or bacterial infection

There is some evidence that a viral infection of the hair follicles could be causing alopecia, and it has been suggested that HIV infection could be a trigger in its onset. Others suggest that a general viral or bacterial infection may lead the immune system to be dysfunctional and then act against the hair follicles in susceptible people. Unfortunately, the evidence for all of these hypotheses is inconsistent.

Hormones

There is clear evidence of a link between pregnancy and alopecia, and there are many reported cases of alopecia in women in the late stages of pregnancy. But women who already have alopecia when they become pregnant may find they have temporary hair regrowth around the time of the birth. Other evidence suggests a link between alopecia and periods of hormonal change – such as puberty and the menopause.

Allergies

There is some evidence that Caucasians (e.g. most white people) with alopecia and some forms of allergic reactions, such as asthma, eczema or rhinitis, have more hair loss than other racial groups.

Chemicals

There have been reports of increased rates of alopecia after exposure to certain kinds of chemicals. For instance, workers at a water treatment plant in a paper factory had high levels of alopecia after they were exposed to the chemical acrylamide. Other chemicals linked to alopecia include formaldehyde and various pesticides. However, there are no *proven* links. Researchers have reported connections between alopecia and medical treatments such as zidovudine (a drug used in the treatment of HIV) and fluvoxamine (an antidepressant drug), but it is difficult to establish whether the alopecia is *caused* by the treatment or is linked in some other way to the disorder. For instance, we do know that alopecia may be associated with depression.

Seasonal changes

You may find that your hair tends to grow back during the summer months, and is lost again during winter. How this might be linked to moulting in animals is not really known. There may also be an association with exposure to UV light.

Is alopecia linked to other diseases?

There have been a number of studies looking at how people with alopecia often have other problems as well. When you read this, though, do not start to panic! The associations are generally very small. Researchers have compared the frequency of a particular disease in a group of people with alopecia with a group of people who do not have alopecia. The differences found are usually small, but they may tell us something about the nature of the condition.

We have already mentioned how it is common to also have problems with fingernails, but associations have also been found with various types of thyroid disease, such as simple goitre, myxoedema and Grave's disease. There are also links with vitiligo, systemic lupus erythematosus, coeliac disease, ulcerative colitis, rheumatoid arthritis, pernicious anaemia, Addison's disease, Legionnaires' Disease, and some ocular and testicular abnormalities. Again, though, it does need to be emphasized that if you have alopecia it does not mean that you will go on to develop these other illnesses.

Now if, after reading this, you are feeling even worse than you did before, you can be cheered by the evidence that alopecia seems to protect against diabetes mellitus. One study comparing alopecia sufferers and their siblings (without alopecia) showed that diabetes was more prevalent in the siblings.

4

Stress

What is the relationship between alopecia and stress?

In 1944, among the Allied troops, there was a large increase in the number of cases of alopecia areata in the weeks prior to D-Day, when the Allied forces were preparing to invade Europe during the Second World War. Research has shown that a large proportion of people with alopecia have a history of stress or anxiety prior to their hair loss, although other studies have *not* found a link between prior stress and alopecia. These inconsistencies, though, may relate to different research designs, and the difficulty of defining stress and understanding the different impact it has on people. Stress is not something that can be objectively measured – it is subjective, and it is this subjective interpretation that is important.

Jenny and Sheila
Jenny and Sheila are sisters, and were both happily married with children. When they learned that their father had been diagnosed with a terminal illness, they reacted very differently. Their father lived alone, and was having problems looking after himself. Sheila – with the support of her husband – devoted herself to her father, visiting his house every day, cooking him a meal, cleaning, and taking him to his hospital appointments. Jenny, though, could not cope with the news. She would not talk to anyone about her feelings, not even her husband, and she cried whenever she saw her father. Several weeks after the news, Jenny's hair started to fall out. This made the situation even worse, and she became clinically depressed.

As we have already seen, the relationship between alopecia and stress is a difficult one to understand. Someone who experiences stress in his or her life may get alopecia as a result; alternatively, someone with alopecia is likely to experience more stress! Thus alopecia can be both a cause and a consequence of stress. While most of the evidence suggests that there *is* a link between stress and the onset of alopecia, there is contradictory evidence. One study found that while the majority of a sample of people with alopecia reported a stressful event in the previous six months, none reported that episodes of hair loss coincided with stressful events. The researchers therefore concluded that the study did not provide evidence of emotional stress playing a significant role in alopecia. The problem with this conclusion is that the stressful event may not lead to *immediate* hair loss. So we need to examine how stress and alopecia are linked – the delay may occur because of a biological mechanism that we do not understand. For this reason, it is important to try to understand the underlying biology of stress, the immune system, and the way the hair works.

What do we mean by 'stress'?

'Stress' is a badly overused word in our society. Originally stress was an engineering term used in relation to the weight a structure such as a bridge could take before breaking. During the twentieth century, though, this has been analogized to the human condition.

How much of a difficult environment can we endure before we break? A stressor is the object (person, job, social conditions) in the environment that is causing the difficulty, and the stress response is the feeling we get when exposed to that object. This can lead to further responses – such as illnesses that may be the result of exposure to the stressor. Many researchers do not believe that we can develop a general model of psychological stress that will explain what factors in the environment lead to problems. This is partly because of the very loose definitions that are used.

To understand psychological stress we must look at how we interpret stressful events and how we cope. We cope best when we have the personal resources and support from family and friends to enable us to deal with the situation. As we saw with Jenny and Sheila, people interpret the same event differently. We become distressed when there is an imbalance between the pressures placed on us in the environment (the stressful event), and our own coping resources. Whether there is a resulting problem depends at least in part on how we view the situation, and this is where personality plays a part.

We can *learn* to think about stressful situations differently, and so deal with them more effectively. If we can change the way we think about events, and develop our coping resources, then we will be able to cope better with environmental stress – and hence be less likely to get a stress-related illness (such as alopecia). (We shall further explore the relationship between stress and coping in Chapter 8.)

Unfortunately, the term 'stress' is now used so loosely in our society that it has become almost meaningless. We are now all 'under stress'. We have stressful jobs; it is stressful to bring up children; stressful to go shopping; stressful to drive in traffic jams, stressful . . . you get the picture! Stress is a major feature of modern life. If we are *all* under stress, how can we determine whether there is a genuine relationship between difficulties in life and alopecia?

How stressed are you?

There is a range of measures used to examine why people become stressed, and they look at different types of stress. One widely used measure involves looking at the number of life events a person has experienced recently. By 'life event' we mean the kinds of things that happen that often cause distress. While this is a very crude measure – after all, we all respond differently to events – it does help people to identify where their stress originates. The second type of measure involves what could be called 'daily hassles'. These are things that are not particularly stressful in themselves, but are the sort of everyday events which, if they occur too often or for a protracted period, might begin to make someone feel stressed.

These simple approaches in assessing stress involve adding up a number of factors/events and determining the amount of stress you are experiencing. The ten most serious life events and daily hassles are listed in Table 1. By 'most serious' we mean that people are provided with a list and then asked to rate how stressful such events are. The ratings are based on an average score.

Life events	Daily hassles
1 Death of spouse	1 Not enough time
2 Divorce	2 Too many things to do
3 Marital separation	3 Troubling thoughts about the future
4 Prison term	4 Too many interruptions
5 Death of close family member	5 Misplacing or losing things
6 Personal injury or illness	6 Health of a family member
7 Marriage	7 Social obligations
8 Fired at work	8 Concerns about standards
9 Marital reconciliation	9 Concerns about getting ahead
10 Retirement	10 Too many responsibilities

Table 1 Life events and daily hassles that cause stress.

Take a look at the lists in Table 1 and think about whether there were particular life events that preceded your alopecia. Perhaps there were events that are not included in the list? Also, think about whether you had, or have, a high level of daily hassles in your life at the time you got alopecia. These may indicate a possibility that there is a link between stress and your alopecia – though it is not possible to be certain about this.

Sally
Sally was happily married and had a good job, but in the course of less than two years she lost everything. She found out her husband was having an affair, so she threw him out of the house. The divorce proceedings were very messy, and Sally's work was seriously affected. While her boss was sympathetic for a few months, her work became so bad that she was eventually dismissed. It was then that Sally noticed her hair had started to fall out.

One area that has received relatively little attention is the relation-ship between 'traumatic stress' as a cause (and possible consequence) of alopecia. Traumatic stress refers to an event that is potentially life-threatening (to self or others) and is likely to induce fear or horror in most people. Traumatic events include war, sexual abuse, disasters, road accidents, etc. It can also include the death of loved ones. When someone experiences a traumatic event they might experience a range of physical and psychological symptoms. These symptoms, if all are present, can mean that someone may be classified as having post-traumatic stress disorder (PTSD). PTSD is characterized by:

- *Re-experiencing the event* – perhaps through being unable to think of anything except the event, or dreaming about it at night, or feeling as though you are still in the situation.
- *Avoidance and emotional numbing*. At the same time as experiencing traumatic memories a person with PTSD tries to avoid thinking about the event. They might avoid going to the place where the event happened. When the memory comes to mind, they try and do other activities that take their minds off it. They may also experience emotional numbing. This occurs when a person has experienced such awful emotions (fear, helplessness, horror) as a result of the event that they stop themselves (involuntarily) from being able to experience *any* emotions – including positive emotions such as love and happiness. This arises because of a fear of experiencing the awful emotions.
- *Physiological hyperarousal*. This set of physical symptoms might include a 'startle reaction', e.g. jumping at the slightest sound. It can also involve sleep difficulties.

For someone to be classified as having PTSD they must not only experience the above symptoms, but these must affect their working, social or family life. And the symptoms must be present for at least one month.

One of the other consequences of experiencing a traumatic event can be alopecia. The immune system can be damaged by stress, particularly by traumatic stress, and this can lead to alopecia in people who are already susceptible.

The next problem, of course, might be that as a consequence of getting alopecia the alopecia itself can act as a traumatic stressor for some people. Clearly, this complicates things! For example, a person can be traumatized by, say, a road accident, and as a consequence of this they get alopecia. Then the alopecia itself becomes a traumatic event, causing further disturbance.

Longer-term effects of stress

Stress can have adverse effects on many physiological systems, and the capacity to deal with stress reduces with age. Repeated stress leads to repeated secretion of stress hormones that can result in damage to the brain in regions that are important for memory.

Stress is linked to our most primitive biological pathways, namely, the nervous, inflammatory and immune systems. Once activated, the animal prepares to deal with a threat by mounting an inflammatory and analgesic response to deal with the possible ensuing infection, pain, and ultimately the removal of offending material. The question remains, though, why does hair become 'offending material' in alopecia?

The physiological response

This last part of the chapter contains more detailed information about how the body responds to stress. This is important in trying to understand the relationship between alopecia and stress.

The stress response

The stress response is a defence mechanism used by the body to protect itself from external damage, whether physical or psychological. The 'fight or flight response' is a stress response. If we are threatened with attack, we can either fight or run away. At the time of the threat we can feel bodily changes – the dry mouth, the churning stomach, the sweat, as the body prepares itself for action. The stress response is automatic. We may think we have control over our behaviour, but a lot of the time we do not!

The body's initial reaction to stress is to send messages from the higher cortical centres of the brain (which initially register that a stressful event has occurred) to the limbic system (an evolutionary 'old' area which is responsible for our drives and motivation), resulting in the release of brain chemical messengers (neurotransmitters) such as noradrenaline, serotonin and acetylcholine. These activate areas of the hypothalamus (again in the 'old' brain), which releases corticotrophin releasing factor (CRF). CRF co-ordinates the body's stress response via the nervous system. CRF is implicated not just in the stress response, but also in the inflammatory response (see below), another important bodily defence system, which is important in alopecia. It is thought that CRF is aided in the stress response by substance P, which has been implicated in alopecia.

Substance P is widely distributed in the nervous system. It functions in the central nervous system as a neurotransmitter and is located in areas of the brain important in affecting the response to both physiological and psychological stress. It is linked to other areas related to stress. Evidence from research with animals shows that substance P increases in the amygdala, a small area of the brain, after stress – and we know the amygdala is linked to stress and emotional responses.

Inflammatory response

The inflammatory response (e.g. what happens when you get a cut) is the body's most primitive of protective mechanisms. It is thought that this evolved even before the existence of nervous systems in animals. The stress response evolved from the inflammatory response, and is closely linked to it. Both kinds of response are found in most animals, and both are important in ensuring the well-being of the animal. The inflammatory response is also linked to the production of CRF. Psychological stressors can, like the stress response, invoke the inflammatory response. This has immediate advantages in situations where tissue damage occurs (such as when fighting), as the inflammatory response will help deal with any such damage or any infections caused by such damage. Furthermore, the immune system evolved from the inflammatory response and is, as we have seen, implicated in alopecia.

How does stress cause alopecia?

If an environmental stressor can cause alopecia, then this must be associated with the physical changes that indicate stress.

A release of the major stress hormones can make the body respond in a similar way to how it reacts to infection or injury. There can be an inflammatory response, which is linked to alopecia.

CRF and substance P initiate the stress response by activating neural pathways in the nervous and hormonal systems, and by releasing stress hormones. These, along with the cytokines induced by stress, initiate the acute phase response and the production of certain proteins, essential mediators of inflammation. The inflammatory response is linked to psychological stress, which in humans evolved later. The same substances mediate both stress and inflammation.

The central nervous system has the capacity to increase and decrease inflammatory changes in response to trauma, infection and stress. Repeated episodes of stress may produce chronic inflammatory changes, which may result in chronic inflammatory problems such as alopecia.

There is an excess of substance P in the scalp of people with alopecia, and substance P is known to accelerate the onset of hair growth. It is greatly increased after depilation in both humans and mice! It may also have a protective role. Another neuropeptide, calciton-gene-related protein (CGRP), has also been linked to alopecia, and reductions in CGRP occur in follicles affected by alopecia. CGRP inhibits antigen presentation, so reduced concentrations could enhance an immunological mechanism. Overall, scientists are still not clear about the full role of these substances.

So what can we conclude about stress and alopecia?

As usual, there is still a lot of research to be carried out in order to understand the link between stress and alopecia, but clearly something is going wrong with the stress response system. This may be linked to individual characteristics such as personality and coping; or it may be related to modern life. In the past, when we were threatened by events in the environment, we responded physically – i.e. we attacked or we fled. In modern industrial societies, we often do not have the means to respond physically, so the stress hormones stay in the body, trying to keep it in readiness for action that never comes. Over the long term this might have serious physical consequences.

Beverley

Beverley, a middle-aged woman with alopecia, suggests that there may be a stress-related cause. 'I believe that it was my body's way of telling me that it has been running on overdrive for a long period of time. Friends say that I have had quite a lot to put up with over the last few years. I would probably put the cause of my alopecia down to the way my body has reacted to a large amount of stress and adrenaline overkill.'

5

Seeking medical help

What is the role of the doctor in dealing with alopecia?

The first thing you might do when unexpectedly starting to lose your hair is to go to your GP, but remember that the family doctor is a generalist, not a specialist, and often is not qualified to provide appropriate treatment for alopecia. Your GP will readily identify the problem, and will ask questions to identify the probable cause, but it is likely that he or she will refer you to a specialist – a dermatologist, who is an expert in skin disorders and who will be able to provide advice on the most appropriate treatment.

Alternatively, if there are psychological issues, your GP may refer you to a clinical psychologist, psychiatrist or counsellor, who will provide appropriate therapy and assistance with psychological problems. The problem with this is that it can be very difficult obtaining this type of therapy. Your GP may be loath to refer you for psychological help for something like hair loss; and even if you are referred, you may have to wait a long time to actually get an appointment.

What is the role of the dermatologist in alopecia?

Unfortunately, most dermatologists are not trained in psychology, so they may not recognize the psychological problems alopecia can bring. They may focus on treating the medical disorder at the expense of not appreciating the psychological problems. There are cases where dermatologists have done more harm than good simply because they have failed to recognize how a person with alopecia feels. Indeed, a study published a few years ago that failed to find a close relationship between stress and alopecia concluded that 'the absence of conclusive evidence justifies the more positive statement to alopecia patients that they are not responsible for their disease nor can they influence its course'. This is a rather disturbing sentence, which attempts to justify a strong medical position, one in which you, the sufferer, are helpless in the face of hair loss, and so need to rely on the 'expertise' of the medical profession. We hope that by the end of this book, even if you have not seen your hair grow, you will realize that you *can* do something – either to help your hair grow or, at the very least, to find ways for you to take responsibility for adapting to living with alopecia.

James
'When I was first sent to a dermatologist I went in wearing my cap. This man, a traditional doctor in his fifties and a white coat, greeted me curtly and ripped off my cap without permission. At that point I was very self-conscious, and was wearing the cap all the time in public. I would not dream of taking it off in front of anyone. My experience of alopecia was only a few months old and I was not yet ready to face the world. This was the point at which I realized that doctors were not going to help me.'

This story related by James is unfortunately all too common, for in our own research we have found many stories of the failure of the medical community to take alopecia seriously. To many doctors, it is simply a dermatological problem. The difficulty may be that doctors generally, and dermatologists especially, may not be aware of the potential psychological impact of alopecia. However, that is not to say there are no sympathetic dermatologists around. We do believe that the situation is improving, and that doctors are becoming more aware of the problems faced by people with alopecia; and that for the sufferer it is much more than a dermatological problem.

Diagnosis – what the dermatologist might tell you

In medical terms there is no conclusive diagnostic test for alopecia. As we explained earlier, scientists are not sure whether alopecia is a single disorder or a set of related but different disorders. A medical diagnosis usually proceeds by the doctor identifying a set of symptoms that constitute a specific disorder, for which there is (hopefully) a known and effective treatment. Unfortunately, alopecia does not fit this pattern, so doctors are faced with a very difficult

38

task. Alopecia has a number of different causes, and so while the main symptom – hair loss – is universal, different causes may require different treatments.

Your dermatologist will attempt to work out whether you have alopecia by eliminating other possibilities and by examining the lesion. As we have seen, alopecia appears at different rates for different people, and has a greater or lesser effect – i.e. it might only be a small patch on the scalp, or it might cover the whole body. A typical case (though bearing in mind that nothing is 'typical' – which is why alopecia is so difficult to diagnose) might involve a bald patch appearing in a 24-hour period. This is usually (but not always) on the scalp. A dermatologist might try a hair pull test at the margins of the affected area. If your hair comes out easily, that indicates alopecia, and it is likely you will experience further hair loss.

Hair fibre taken from this point can be sent for analysis. Observing the hair under an electron microscope will show that the hair is unusual. The part of the hair furthest from the scalp (the older part) looks normal, but the shape becomes irregular nearer to the scalp. This includes deposits of keratin (the protein that makes up the hair), and also constrictions in the fibre of the hair. There are often cracks along the hair. The difference from a normal hair lies not in the amount of keratin present, but in the way it is assembled.

These hair fibres can have weak spots that lead to breakage. Sometimes the stump of the hair looks like an exclamation mark. This is very distinctive in alopecia, and the dermatologist might look for this as one of the signs of alopecia – noting, of course, that such hair can appear in other conditions as well!

We have already seen how a further sign of alopecia is problems with fingernails. It is difficult to work out how many people have this problem, and it does not always occur at the same time as the onset of alopecia, but somewhere between 10 per cent and 30 per cent of people with alopecia have such a problem – it depends which reports you read! Nails may become pitted, their growth may be affected, or they may be very soft.

Another diagnostic technique used by dermatologists involves carrying out a skin biopsy. This involves taking a small piece of skin (about 4 mm in diameter) and examining it under the microscope. The dermatologist can then see whether there is focal inflammation of the hair follicles, which is one of the clearest signs of alopecia.

There is a possibility that this could be done using blood samples instead, but as yet there is no accepted technique for doing so.

Other professionals who can provide help

It is important that any medical practitioner who is dealing with cases of alopecia determines whether there are any associated psychological or social problems. If there are, they will need to be dealt with appropriately. Such issues may include anything from marriage problems to work-related stress. Dealing with such associated problems may lead to a better outcome for the alopecia. The possibilities vary according to what is available in your area, but your GP should be able to refer you to a clinical psychologist or a psychiatrist for help with any psychological problems you may have. (The kinds of techniques that they employ are described in Chapter 8.)

What is the difference between a clinical psychologist,
a psychiatrist, a psychotherapist and a counsellor?

In the UK, a clinical psychologist normally has a psychology degree, followed by three years of further training that will prepare them for a range of treatment strategies with a variety of mental illnesses. Sometimes a GP's clinic may have a clinical psychologist who does a number of sessions a week at the practice, but it is more likely that you will be referred to a hospital for outpatient treatment – and there is often a long wait for this. Clinical psychologists cannot prescribe drugs.

A psychiatrist is a medical doctor, who has done a medical degree, and has then trained to specialize in mental health. A psychiatrist can prescribe drugs, and apply a range of psychological methods.

A psychotherapist is someone who provides therapy. They may be any one of the above, or – more likely – someone trained in specific kinds of therapies used to treat particular problems. The level of training varies dramatically.

The term 'counsellor' is used very broadly, generally referring to someone who is more of a listener than a therapist.

A much quicker way of getting treatment is to use a counsellor. Again, more and more GP clinics have counsellors at their surgeries, but counsellors can be found in many places. There are different types of counsellors. Some are better trained than others, and there are a variety of different techniques that they use. If you are thinking of using a counsellor you need to ensure that they are going to offer you a treatment that is right for you. (See Further Information at the back of this book.)

People with alopecia also use alternative practitioners such as trichologists (who specialize in the treatment of hair), homeopaths, acupuncturists, and others.

6

Available treatments

What are the options?

In ancient Egypt, people would cover their baldness with a mixture of fats from ibex, lions, crocodiles, serpents, geese and hippopotami. How effective this was we cannot say – there are no records. Julius Caesar took another approach – he covered his balding head with laurels. It has been suggested that the ceremonial use of a laurel wreath stems from Caesar's vanity!

There are a lot of myths surrounding treatment for hair loss. Standing on your head to increase the blood flow to the brain will not cure it, nor is there any evidence that massaging your scalp helps – though this might help you relax, which itself could lead to hair regrowth.

There is a range of medical treatments available. As we said in an earlier chapter, these may be effective, at least temporarily, with the milder forms of alopecia, but rarely work if you have alopecia totalis or universalis. We cannot present you with any clear conclusions about what will work in which circumstances. In the end, all treatments are palliative – i.e. they can help to control the problem, but they rarely cure it. Even if you have patchy alopecia areata it is questionable whether the treatments themselves are effective or whether you would recover anyway without treatment. Because of these problems, and because some of the treatments may be painful or have side-effects, having any form of treatment should involve an informed choice.

There are several factors to be taken into account regarding the potential for hair regrowth. Such regrowth is less likely if:

- The alopecia is more serious (totalis or universalis).
- It starts before 16 years of age.
- Nails are affected.
- There is rapid progression.
- The hair loss takes place over a period of months rather than days or weeks.

There is no conclusive evidence that medical treatments alter the ultimate course of the disease. If you are developing alopecia universalis, then there is no known treatment to stop this occurring. Neither has any treatment been conclusively shown to do anything more than suppress the active immunological process. Because of this, only long-term treatment will have any long-term effect; because once the treatment stops, the immunological system is again activated and hair loss is likely to resume. Treatments often have side-effects, and these must be weighed against any cosmetic benefits.

Drug treatments should usually last at least three months before an assessment can be made of their effectiveness. If you have alopecia areata it may be necessary to treat unaffected areas of the scalp as well as affected areas, because these may develop an inflammatory reaction and lead to further hair loss. Doctors may also recommend leaving an affected area untreated to check the degree of spontaneous hair regrowth.

It may be possible to increase the chances of hair regrowth through the use of more than one drug at the same time. This technique is used, but has not been assessed scientifically to see whether it has a beneficial effect. The danger of this approach is that there may be side-effects not only from each drug, but also from the combination of drugs – and the effects here are not known.

Beware!

There are endless ideas being marketed by the medical community, alternative practitioners and those within the cosmetics industry, which, it is claimed, will lead to hair regrowth. The proliferation of these treatments is indicative of the number of people who are very concerned about their hair. If a treatment is discovered that is effective with all forms of alopecia, we will soon know about it. It is almost a search for the Holy Grail. If something is found it will be on the front page of every newspaper and on the radio and television news headlines!

Types of treatment

Topical corticosteroids

These are creams that are rubbed into the scalp. There is limited evidence regarding their efficacy. They may work when someone has patchy alopecia, but they do not work with people who have alopecia totalis or alopecia universalis. For instance, one randomized control trial with 70 patients with patchy alopecia using desoximetasone cream indicated a trend in the treatment group to have more hair regrowth, but the effect was not significantly greater than in the placebo group.

Minoxidil (sold as Rogaine)

This is one of the most widely used treatments for alopecia, and is used only in adults. There is some evidence of limited effectiveness in some individuals, but it is unlikely to lead to full recovery of hair. One study showed that after four months of treatment, 59 per cent of men and women experienced at least some hair regrowth. Twenty-six per cent had moderate to dense hair growth, the rest minimal growth. One of the problems is that even if there is some regrowth, the individual cannot stop using minoxidil because the hair is likely to fall out again. Many doctors are sceptical about the benefits, observing only the growth of vellus hair, which is light and fuzzy, rather than normal hair. Minoxidil may also lead to side-effects such as an itchy scalp. Furthermore, it only seems to benefit the crown of the head, not the front.

Minoxidil appears to have a direct stimulating effect on the hair follicle, prolonging the anagen (growth) phase. However, the evidence for any effect on the immune system is controversial. Minoxidil has a number of side-effects, such as headaches, dizziness, itching, allergic reactions and heartbeat irregularities.

Dithranol (sold as Micanol)

This has also been found to have some effect, with at least some hair regrowth in around two-thirds of patients. Dithranol can be applied as a cream either to the entire scalp or to specific areas of hair loss. If the former, then treatment should start with a localized area and exposure gradually increased. One of the side-effects can be staining of the hair and scalp. It may also be irritating to the skin. If the

44

person has light-coloured hair, this can be a significant problem. It is thought that dithranol has an impact on immune function.

Minoxidil has been used in combination with dithranol, so there can be a combined effect on immune function and on prolonging the anagen phase of the hair follicle. Some dermatologists believe their effects are additive because of these different modes of action. One side-effect is facial hair growth, but this may be due to accidental application to the face.

Topical treatment is one of the most promising ways forward, but inevitably there are potential problems. It is possible that some substances are carcinogenic (can cause cancer).

Injecting corticosteroids

Injecting corticosteroids directly into the scalp is thought to be the most effective treatment for alopecia. It can be used to treat patchy hair loss and for areas the individual has particular problems with, such as eyebrows.

Generally speaking, for people with patchy alopecia areata, around two-thirds of patients will respond to corticosteroids injected into the scalp. Multiple scalp injections are given by the dermatologist every four to six weeks.

Two commonly used substances are hydrocortisone acetate and triamcinolone acetonide. The corticosteroid is injected into the skin. Several injections may need to be given, and this will probably be uncomfortable for the patient. The other problem is that if someone receives several injections in the same area, it can cause skin problems. There is also a risk of cataract when injecting close to the eyes.

Between injections, maintenance therapy may be given with topical corticosteroids, such as betamethasone diproprionate cream (0.05%), applied twice daily.

Systemic corticosteroids

Corticosteroids (anti-inflammatory steroids) have been used for many years to treat dermatologic disorders, including alopecia, and daily treatment with oral corticosteroids will produce some hair regrowth in some people. One study showed that 30–47 per cent of patients treated with prednisolone showed at least 25 per cent hair regrowth. The drawback is that the treatment needs to be prolonged.

Other studies also show some benefit in the use of oral corticosteroids for people with limited alopecia. The problem with the research is that there are not enough good randomized controlled studies, and so it is difficult to compare treatment effectiveness with spontaneous remission.

Systemic corticosteroids have also been used with those who have rapidly progressing and more extensive alopecia. They may reduce active hair loss, but – yet again – hair loss may recur once treatment stops. The use of systemic corticosteroids has significant risks as the drug is being taken orally, and there may be a medical impact in other areas of the body. Prolonged or excessive use can lead to systemic levels that produce undesirable side-effects, such as salt retention or suppression of the function of the pituitary and adrenal glands. There may also be inappropriate hair growth or weight gain. In the longer term, the use of corticosteroids may contribute to osteoporosis.

Contact immunotherapy

There is a possibility that alopecia can be treated through biological therapy, or immunotherapy, in which the body's own cells or chemicals are used to help boost the natural immune response against the disorder. This is a technique used in cancer treatment. However, with both alopecia and cancer, there is little evidence that the approach works.

Gene therapy

Your combination of genes is a matter of luck – we do not get to choose our parents! (Nor do our children get to choose us!) In the past there was little that could be done about our genetic inheritance. Today, though, techniques are being developed that can implant genes that alter biological characteristics. Gene therapy for hair regrowth is in its infancy, but has potential for the future.

Knowledge about the genetic defects that lead to alopecia suggests that alopecia can be treated by altering these altered genes. One strategy is to replace a defective gene with its normal counterpart, using methods of recombinant DNA technology. Researchers still need to develop methods that can be used to insert genes into normal hair cells, though.

The reality at the moment, though, is that you will not obtain a cure for alopecia through gene therapy.

Surgery

Only a couple of decades ago, if someone had a hair transplant they would almost inevitably end up looking a mess. Fortunately, things have improved. There are basically two techniques in use: transplantation and scalp reduction.

It is not surprising that people with alopecia feel so terrible that they are prepared to consider surgery. Hair transplant surgery has been around for several decades; it has usually been cosmetic surgery, used on men with common baldness. Techniques have been refined over the years and surgeons can now make a good job of transplanting hair. The problem, though, is when the area affected is very large. The cost of a hair transplant is linked to the size of area that has to be operated on. The greater the hair loss, the greater the cost – and you cannot get it on the NHS. A further problem is that if you have lost *all* the hair on your head, transplantation is unlikely to be feasible.

If you are going to consider hair transplantation it is important to ensure that you use a reputable surgeon. Unfortunately, the vanity brigade has made huge inroads into this area and special offers abound in magazines and on the high street. It is essential to take the advice of your GP and your dermatologist if you are thinking about a transplant.

A further problem is that hair transplants can have side-effects. The resulting scarring on the skin can be serious, and the area is also more likely to become infected.

If the above does not put you off, then you should be aware of the different kinds of transplant available. There are various terms used – including hair grafting, punch grafting, plug grafting, or hair transplantation. It involves taking small pieces of hair-bearing scalp from the back and sides of the head and moving them into slits and holes on the top of the head. Some specific terms include:

Micrografting
This is the most sophisticated form of transplant. One or two hairs are individually implanted into the skin on the head (a bit like potting plants). This can give a natural appearance, but it is also the most time-consuming and expensive form of transplantation.

Small or large slit grafts
This involves putting three or four small hairs, or six or seven large hairs, in a slit recipient hole.

Small or large minigraft
This involves putting three or four small hairs, or between five and eight large hairs, into a recipient site.

Flap grafting
A skin graft is taken from one area and transplanted to another. The graft, containing intact follicles, is often taken from the back of the head. The flap remains attached at one end. It obtains its nourishment through this, so the hair in the flap will continue to grow normally. This technique transfers the most hair in the shortest time, but the surgery is extensive and you will need a highly skilled and experienced surgeon.

There are other forms of surgery available:

Scalp reduction
This involves inserting devices under the skin to stretch the areas of scalp that still have hair; the redundant bald areas are then removed. Usually, several sites are stretched. The success of the operation will depend on the flexibility of the scalp, the degree of hair loss, and the age of the person. Most scalp reductions also include flaps or grafts.

Hair stitching
This involves implanting artificial hair fibres into the scalp.

> *Important note*: Remember, if you intend to have any form of surgery, ensure that you obtain appropriate advice. Talk to your GP and your dermatologist – they will offer advice regarding what is best for you. If surgery is an option, they will recommend an appropriately skilled and experienced surgeon.

Hair weaving

This involves weaving pieces of hair into the person's already existing hair. It is woven tightly into the existing hair, so tightly that it might cause traction alopecia – that is, the hair could be pulled out. This technique can be particularly devastating for someone with alopecia areata, because the hairs around the bald patches tend to be loose and hence can be pulled out more easily.

Wigs

Wearing a wig is the most common option for many people with alopecia. In Britain wigs can be obtained on the NHS (though you still have to make a contribution to the price), and can be made to match any style or colour. Wigs vary dramatically in quality. Some are made of real hair, some are artificial. As with most things, the more you are willing to pay the better quality the hairpiece, and the more realistic it looks. Many people are very happy with their wigs, though there are a number of problems associated with them – they can be very hot to wear, and they might blow off in the wind (though they can be fastened down).

Wigs provide some advantages to those who wear them. Wig-wearers do not have to appear bareheaded, and so they reduce anxiety. Also, wigs enable the wearer to choose how they look. They are flexible, because style and colour can be varied. On the other hand, some people, particularly women, may find it difficult to take them off, even at home, or with their partner/husband.

If we can extend the concept of cure to include wigs, they are probably the most effective 'cure' for some people, as wigs allow people to go out in public looking (and feeling) 'normal'.

Tattooing

Tattooing is used by some people with alopecia totalis or universalis to replace eyelashes and eyebrows that have been lost. The loss of hair from the face can profoundly affect the sense of identity, so tattooing new eyebrows can provide psychological relief. If you are going to consider a tattoo, then you need to think carefully. A badly done tattoo can be a permanent problem for you, and if it is on your face it will be much worse. You should discuss this option with your doctor, and find a reputable tattooist, preferably via recommendation from other people with alopecia who have already been tattooed. You can contact other people with alopecia via several websites (see Further Information at the back of this book).

Complementary therapies

Many people with alopecia turn to complementary therapies to find a way of making their hair grow again. There are various complementary therapies available, such as homeopathy, herbalism, hypnotherapy and food supplements. There is little evidence that they have any medical value, but that is not to say they do not have psychological value. Certain forms of complementary therapy may help you relax, and hence feel better in yourself. There is also the problem in that only certain types of people are likely to consider using complementary therapies, and these are the people who are most likely to think them effective, so there may be a placebo effect.

The medical community is ambivalent about complementary therapies. Many medical practitioners reject them out of hand; others embrace them. The evidence for the effectiveness of such treatments is at best weak, but, like traditional medical treatments, this is not necessarily a good reason to reject them. It may be best for some people to combine traditional medical treatments with alternative therapies.

Herbal treatments are fairly popular for a range of dermatological conditions. The Chinese claim that hair loss is related to weakness in the liver or kidneys or a deficiency in the blood. Herbs that will help nourish these organs and the blood should remedy this. The problem with some of the Chinese herbal creams is that they can be adulterated with corticosteroids, so it might be difficult to establish which is having an effect – the herb or the steroid! One study showed 8 out of 11 such creams contained steroids. Herbal medicines can also have side-effects; and if you have other immune disorders, these may be exacerbated by the use of steroids.

Hypnotherapy is often used and it can be effective. This is one area where helping the person with alopecia to relax may be beneficial in itself.

So should you use complementary therapies?

This is a controversial area. Scientists are not in agreement about whether complementary therapies are effective; and neither are they in agreement about which ones are the most effective. One study found that rubbing essential oils into the scalp encouraged hair growth, so aromatherapy may be an effective treatment. In the end, we just don't know how well these therapies work; and whether or not you use them depends on your own circumstances. At the very least, many of the treatments are very relaxing – itself something that is much appreciated if you have alopecia!

If these therapies work only to the extent that they reduce stress and enhance well-being, then they are beneficial.

Treatment for other problems related to your alopecia

As we have seen, it is possible that you not only have a problem with alopecia, but perhaps also psychological disorders such as depression and anxiety. Your GP will be in a position to advise you regarding treatments for these conditions. Apart from psychological therapies offered by psychologists (which are described elsewhere in the book), you may be offered medication. You should always take care over any decision regarding medication for psychological problems such as depression and anxiety, because they may simply mask the symptoms, and when you come off the drugs the symptoms may return. Some treatments may also be addictive. On the other hand, if you are having severe difficulties in your daily living because of these problems, then it may be wise to take some form of medication so that you can handle your everyday life.

Any medication for such problems must be considered in relation to any drug treatments you are undergoing for the alopecia, because there is always the danger of both side-effects and also an interaction between the effects of the two drugs.

There are various kinds of treatment available. There are a range of standard anti-anxiety and antidepressant drugs; for instance, imipramine (tricyclic antidepressant), doxepine (sedative antidepressant with anxiolytic action), and alprazolam (triazolobenzodiazapine with slight antidepressive action). One type of newer and effective treatment is using SSRIs, or serotonin-specific reuptake inhibitors. Prozac is the best known example of this type of antidepressant. In recent years these drugs have been widely prescribed for a variety of anxiety and depressive illnesses. Recent research indicates that these drugs may have unpleasant side-effects and may well be addictive. Any decision to take them should be fully discussed with your GP.

It is not known what effect any of these drugs may have on the course of your alopecia. It is possible that the use of anxiety- and depression-relieving drugs may help with hair growth, but as yet there is no evidence either way.

51

Conclusions with regard to treatment

There are always new treatments coming on the market. Some of these are simply quack medicines, which gain popularity because people with alopecia are desperate to find something that will make their hair grow back and are willing to try anything. There are ever-increasing numbers of drugs available, which are constantly being tested for efficacy. As we have seen, the evidence for the drugs we have so far is limited, to say the least. We do not believe that treatment for alopecia has advanced much beyond creating substances that might delay hair loss, or might lead to some limited improvement in the more minor cases of alopecia. There is as yet no wonder cure, nor is there one on the horizon.

If your alopecia is patchy and limited to the head you have a fair chance of recovery, though there will always be the threat of recurrence; some drugs can provide limited help for you.

If your alopecia is totalis or universalis, or you have had the alopecia with little or no regrowth, then there are no drugs available that will guarantee hair regrowth. That is a fact, and something that you must accept. There may be a treatment available in the future, but there is nothing now.

For some people there is the possibility of hair transplantation, but this is only viable if you have hair to transplant. It is not for totalis or universalis patients. For others, wigs and tattoos are useful cosmetics.

One study has examined the effects of using a combination of treatment strategies with alopecia patients. The treatments included the use of a strong immunosuppressant, and at the same time the people in the study were taught relaxation and image therapy. There was some evidence of effectiveness as nearly all of the patients who tried relaxation combined with the drugs had some hair regrowth. This suggests that relief from stress facilitates the recovery of the immune system.

The overall view appears rather pessimistic, but there are positive signs. Gene therapy is likely to provide an effective cure within the next few years – but is not available yet. Also, new drugs are constantly coming on to the market. The more we understand the causes of alopecia, the closer we come to an effective treatment. Advances are certainly being made in understanding how and why alopecia occurs, but these advances are not yet sufficient to supply guaranteed cures.

This is the reason why most of the rest of the book is taken up with *dealing with* alopecia. If you have alopecia, particularly the more serious forms, then you need to learn how to deal with it, how to adapt to having no hair, how to manage your life, your family, your work, and how to cope with stress. The good news is that humans are good at adaptation.

7

The impact of alopecia

The personal consequences of alopecia can be utterly devastating, although it is easy to understand why many people who have never suffered hair loss might not understand this. After all, it is only hair. Why should it matter? Many people choose to shave the hair off their heads. Being bald is a statement of style. This naïve view, while understandable, does not even begin to touch on the pain experienced by the many people who do lose their hair. A person who experiences alopecia has not *chosen* to have no hair – they have not made a fashion statement. One day they were happily living in the world with a full head of hair, and the next they are bald – or at least a lot of their hair has fallen out.

Mary
Mary was at university, studying law. She wanted to become a barrister. She always obtained good marks in her exams, she was popular with other students, and was loved by her family. She first noticed a bald spot towards the end of her second year, when she was revising for her exams. For the first few days she thought little of it, but when another patch appeared, and then another, she started to worry. She went to her GP who told her she had alopecia. She immediately logged on to the internet and found out all about it. But her hair continued to fall out, and she became depressed. By the time her exams came round she had taken to wearing a hat in public, as she could no longer cover up the patches. She failed her exams. During the summer her hair grew back and her confidence began to return. She re-sat her exams and continued her studies, but unfortunately the patches started to appear again, and this time there were more of them. Eventually Mary could not face going into lectures and seminars, and she did not complete her studies.

The time course of alopecia

The first thing someone with alopecia wants to know is 'Will my hair grow back?' The second is 'When will it grow back?' The third is 'Will it be normal?' These questions are difficult to answer. As mentioned in an earlier chapter, it is hard to predict what will happen to any given individual. Unfortunately the best answers to these questions are, respectively, 'Don't know', 'It might not', and 'Possibly – but, then again, possibly not'.

A reminder:

- The less hair that has been lost, the more likely it is to grow back.
- People with alopecia totalis and alopecia universalis rarely have full regrowth.
- Once you have experienced alopecia, you are likely to experience it again.
- Hair that does return tends not to grow back properly.

People with alopecia totalis and alopecia universalis are the ones who are most likely to experience both psychological and social difficulties that they need to overcome. The social difficulties will be considered in the next chapter, but the personal factors will be considered here.

Identity change

Helen
'I used to be very proud of my hair. It was almost black, and went down to my waist. Everyone told me how nice it looked. I didn't think about it at the time, but it somehow made me the person I was. After my accident my hair fell out very quickly – it was all gone within a few weeks. When I looked in the mirror the person I saw looking back was not me. It was someone else. It is very difficult to describe what I mean by that, but simply because I do not have any hair I am now a different person; and I behave differently with people. Inside I still remember who I was, but in everything I do, and in most things, I think I am someone else.'

Many people with severe alopecia talk about identity change, about being a different person now they have no hair, yet people around them often dismiss these feelings as silly or ridiculous. If you feel that your identity has changed since you've had alopecia, then do not worry. You are not alone, and it is perfectly normal to have these feelings. In fact, becoming aware of your changed identity is often

55

the first step to psychological recovery. Recognizing that the problem is likely to be permanent – which is what you have done – is the first stage to coping with the future.

What is the 'self'?

We all have a sense of self, of knowing who we are, and we develop our sense of self throughout life. What we are is dependent on a whole range of factors, including personality, genes, family environment, schooling, friends, etc. Self is very important to us, for it provides a sense of who we are and a sense of stability. You probably feel that at one level you are the same person now as you were 20 years ago, but at the same time notions of the self change. While you believe yourself to be the same person, in other ways you know that you have changed, probably in many ways. You might have become a husband or wife, a parent; you might have a new career role, a new hobby, all of which change you. Changes are also brought about by people you meet and interact with; by the books and newspapers you read; by what you hear on the radio. All these factors feed into your memory, and change you. You have thought about them – sometimes unconsciously – and they have changed you.

Simultaneously, therefore, the self is both stable and changing. It determines how you think; it is your sense of being 'me'. We maintain and develop our self-identity through a process of *narrative*. Narrative is story-telling. We are all familiar with story-telling; it is something we experience as children. We read stories in books and in newspapers. It is also how our sense of self develops – as a life story. Under normal circumstances this narrative develops slowly in a fairly predictable fashion. New people come into our lives, they influence us, and our life story develops. But under certain circumstances, our narratives are broken. They are torn apart by some traumatic event: war, rape, death, disaster. These kinds of events destroy what we know about the world – namely, that people are generally kind, and that the world is generally a good place. A person who gets alopecia suddenly realizes that the world is not always a good place. It can hurt. It can also affect relationships, and make you realize that people are not necessarily kind either.

At one level this sounds trivial – surely we all know that people and the world can be terrible places? Of course, but until it happens to us, we do not fully realize the implications of this.

How can alopecia destroy identity?

The sense of self is essential to our equilibrium and well-being. If the sense of self is not stable, then we enter disequilibrium; and alopecia, because it is a fundamental disfigurement, can destabilize our conceptions of self. This is because the self is not just psychological – it is not just about the way we think, it is also about the way we look. From an early age we learn to recognize ourselves, and children as young as two or three will recognize themselves in a mirror. From that point on, our identity is linked to our physical appearance. When we reach adolescence we spend a lot of time working at our appearance – not just clothes, but also hairstyles and, for women, make-up. Physical appearance is important to us at this time (the problems experienced by children and adolescents will be addressed in detail in a later chapter), and we continue to be concerned about our physical appearance as adults. People who look at us *do* judge us by our appearance. That is what they see first, so this is not surprising.

Hair is the key to physical appearance.

Think about what you mean by identity. What factors do you think influence the person you are (physical, emotional, personality, friendships, etc.)? If you have alopecia, think about how these factors influenced you before you had alopecia. Write a list, and next to this list write down how you think these have changed because of your alopecia.

The more the degree of change, the greater the potential for experiencing problems. If you emphasize physical appearance and hair as important – and that is not a shallow view, physical appearance *is* important – then you are more likely to have a problem.

Disfigurement

There has been a great deal of research carried out in the field of facial disfigurement – that is a nasty phrase, and you may wonder what it is doing here. The reason we have used it is that severe alopecia has the same impact as facial disfigurement.

William

'I know that I am a different person since I have had alopecia. That is not a trivial statement, but a statement of what I know to be true about myself. When I had hair I was one person, but when it all fell out I became another. When you lose your eyebrows and eyelashes along with all your hair, you cannot remain the same. You look in a mirror and a stranger stares back. Before the hair loss I knew who I was. Some people thought me good-looking, some did not. Those who did think I was good-looking generally mentioned my thick wavy hair, my full eyebrows, and my long eyelashes. When I lost all that I lost what I thought were my best features. It was a long time before I could look in a mirror, and even now I do not like doing so, because it is still that stranger staring back at me.'

Treating alopecia as a disfigurement disorder is a good starting point, for it recognizes that you – particularly if you have totalis or universalis – look fundamentally different from how you looked before you had alopecia. There is a lot of good advice on the Changing Faces website (see Further Information) about how to deal with facial disfigurement (not from the perspective of alopecia, but that does not matter).

Grieving

One of the first things that happen to many people who experience alopecia is that they grieve for their hair. This is normal. A person who experiences any serious loss is likely to grieve for that loss. Grieving is not reserved for death. It is a series of psychological states we go through when we lose something precious. As we have seen, our hair is precious to most of us. Grieving may involve being angry, depressed, suicidal, emotionally numb and, eventually, at the end of the process, a sense that life continues. That last element is something to remember if you are still grieving for your lost hair.

What problems and issues arise for particular groups?

This section is a bit of a misnomer, for anyone with alopecia is a special case. Its purpose, though, is to explore some of the issues that are important to individuals who belong to particular groups.

We have seen that anyone can get alopecia, whether male or female, young or old; and it is a disorder that is found in most societies at roughly the same rates. The previous chapters have considered alopecia in a fairly general sense, assuming that different groups experience alopecia for similar reasons, that the effects are similar, and that there are personal and social consequences. In this section we look in more detail at specific groups who may have greater difficulties than others with alopecia.

At the outset, alopecia affects everyone differently. It is not appropriate to say that if you belong to such and such a group you are more likely, or less likely, to experience problems. We do not know how we will cope until it happens. Dealing with the personal and social consequences depends, as we have seen, on factors such as personality, coping style and social support. The impact of these factors is unpredictable.

Examining the impact of alopecia at different stages of life is important because life is a developmental process. We are different people at different stages. In order to provide a framework we will use a theory originally proposed some decades ago by Erikson, a developmental psychologist.

We have seen how our identities can be affected by alopecia, how there can be a fundamental breakdown of the self, and how damaging this can be. We can try to put this into perspective. Erikson suggested that there are eight stages of life we all go through, and that during each one there is a 'crisis' that has to be resolved. On resolving these crises, the individual develops a new relationship with the environment. The ways in which we choose to deal with the crises will impact on our lives.

Erikson's life stages
1 Infancy: trust vs mistrust.
2 Early childhood: autonomy vs shame and doubt.
3 Pre-school: initiative vs guilt.
4 School age: industry vs inferiority.
5 Puberty: identity vs identity confusion.
6 Young adulthood: intimacy vs isolation.
7 Middle adulthood: generivity vs stagnation.
8 Late adulthood: ego integrity vs despair.

These stages do vary in importance, and certain crises may be more serious for people who develop alopecia, such as adolescents. The consequences are not just for the particular stage at which a person gets alopecia, but the developmental consequences can be much more far-reaching, particularly if the alopecia occurs at a crisis point in the individual's life. This developmental perspective is crucial if we are going to fully understand the impact of alopecia.

We will look at some of the main stages, and then we will focus on another special group – women. Women tend to have greater difficulty adapting to alopecia than men – certainly in our society. In Western culture, hair is very important for a woman, and it forms a central part of her identity; this is not to deny the same is true of men, but for males a bald head is more acceptable. It still involves a change of identity for men, but it is to a type of identity acceptable in society. A bald head on a woman is not acceptable. This is evidenced by the fact that more women with alopecia wear wigs. (The final section of this chapter is concerned with problems experienced by men.)

What are the problems for children?

Alopecia in children can be a special tragedy. Children with alopecia can suffer terribly from bullying, both physical and verbal. This has a severe emotional impact. Children are well known for their cruelty, for some of them do not have the veneer of civilization that stops older people from being insulting and cruel. Children with alopecia often have a lot of time off school because they are unable to face their peers; they cannot face being out in public. It can be very difficult for children to cope with alopecia.

The role of the school will be very significant for a child with alopecia. It is important that the teachers in the school prepare the other children for the return of a child with alopecia. Teachers can educate, advise, cajole, threaten – whatever is necessary in order to reduce the chances of pupils bullying or otherwise being cruel to the child with alopecia. If this is done effectively, then it dramatically reduces the possibility of bullying. Further support can be provided by the school by ensuring that the child with alopecia always has someone they can turn to if they have problems. The child will in all probability rely quite heavily on their close friends, and there is no need for schools to interfere with this, apart from ensuring that the friends understand the effects of alopecia, and that they are not becoming emotionally disturbed by their experiences with the child with alopecia.

If you are a parent of a child with alopecia you can make a substantial contribution to helping the school prepare for the return of your child. First, you should open a dialogue with the head teacher and class teacher to ensure they are aware of the problems. It is unlikely that the teachers will know much about alopecia, so you can act as a useful source of information. This dialogue should continue through the period of the child's return, to ensure that both parties are aware of any problems that may arise – such as bullying and teasing.

It is important that you are aware of the potential issues for your child, such as bullying, communicating with other parents and children, whether the child wants to wear a wig, and the emotions they may be feeling (anger, frustration, depression, etc.). You should talk to them, spend time with them, emphasize the positive aspects of life, and help them through the inevitable crises that occur. Children will have different needs at different times, and it is important that you are aware of these needs. Work with the school to help minimize bullying and teasing, and encourage the school to inform the other pupils about the problem.

Linda

Linda, an eight-year-old, suddenly lost all her hair. To start with she stayed off school, too upset to attend. To help her back to school the head teacher talked to the children during assembly, emphasizing that Linda was ill, and that the illness had made her lose her hair and she was very upset about it. The head teacher explained about alopecia and told the children that Linda was coming back to school the following week and asked them to help her get better. On her return to school, the head teacher and Linda's parents monitored the situation and there were no serious difficulties. They put it down to the children being involved in helping Linda to get better.

What are the problems for adolescents?

Adolescence involves a crisis of identity versus role confusion.

Adolescents are faced with deciding who and what they want to be in terms of work, beliefs and attitudes, and behaviour patterns. Successful adolescents will find a role for themselves and establish a strong sense of identity; those who do not succeed may become confused and withdrawn.

Adolescents are notoriously unpredictable and emotional. They are passing through a period of identity development, and any emotional crisis can damage this. We have talked throughout this book in terms of the problems with identity that anyone with alopecia might face. These difficulties are inevitably going to be more serious for someone who is actively trying to establish their identity in the first place.

If you experience alopecia during adolescence, then resolving this crisis properly is going to be very difficult. It will be difficult not only with regard to selfhood, but also because this is the time when both boys and girls do their best to make themselves attractive to the opposite sex. To lose one's hair at this stage can have a serious impact on development.

Puberty marks a significant change for young males and females, and major physical changes take place. Our bodies reach maturity, males become capable of impregnating females, and females become capable of bearing children. The onset of puberty varies a lot, beginning as early as 8–10 in girls, and 10–12 in boys, but may not occur until about 15. One of the major changes for both boys and girls is the amount of hair they have. Both sexes grow hair in the pubic regions and under the arms, and increase the amount of hair they have all over their bodies, and boys develop a beard. To experience alopecia at this point can create serious emotional problems, aside from identity issues. Many people – perhaps particularly boys – are concerned that they are progressing properly through puberty. If they find that they are not developing hair appropriately, they may feel inadequate, and if alopecia strikes at this point it can be devastating.

What are the problems for young adults?

According to Erikson, the task facing young adults is to be able to share their lives with another person in a close and committed relationship. Successful people will have intimate relationships, and those who do not succeed will become isolated from others. If you have alopecia, this isolation may be more severe. Friends and family of a young adult with alopecia should ensure they have plenty of support.

By young adults we are referring to people who have passed through puberty and may be embarking on a career. The most serious problems people in work are likely to face relate to not being able to progress because of fears of inadequacy because of alopecia, and this may impede career development. They may also experience relationship problems. This is the stage at which many people are settling into long-term relationships, and are thinking about having children. The onset of alopecia can be very detrimental to this process.

What are the problems for middle-aged adults?

The challenge during this stage of life is to be creative, productive, and to nurture the next generation. Those who succeed in this will be more creative, productive and nurturing; and those who fail will be passive and self-centred, perhaps feeling that the world is not better off because they are alive.

This age group is the time when many people are settling into a new phase of life – one not usually dominated by young children – and they are probably at the peak of their careers. Alopecia may not affect some middle-aged people quite as seriously as those in younger age groups: older people are settled in their identity and often quite strong in knowing the direction their life is taking. They are most likely to be able to afford the best medical treatments and, if necessary, the best wigs. However, it may still impact seriously on people in this age band, who may also be concerned about ageing. If adolescents are in the stage of being embarrassed by their parents and one of those parents experiences alopecia, this can be doubly embarrassing for the teenager – and may harm the relationship between parent and child.

Many women start to experience alopecia from the time of the menopause. This may consist of simple thinning of the hair rather than alopecia areata.

What are the problems in old age?

Many older people experience alopecia. The task at this stage of life is to see whether we can attain wisdom, a sense of wholeness, and acceptance of what life means and has meant (ego integrity versus despair). Older people who succeed here will enjoy life and not fear death. Those who fail will feel that their life is empty and they will be frightened of dying. These may be the people who are more likely to experience alopecia.

What are the problems for women?

Eugenia Ginzburg was a Russian woman transported to the Gulags during the Soviet era. She was sharing a truck with 76 other people when the train stopped near Irkutsk, in Siberia; more women were put on board. These women were suffering starvation and disease, but there was something far worse – their heads had been shaved. This is, for many, the supreme insult to womanhood. Ginzburg says, 'I ran my fingers through my hair. No, that is something I thought I would hardly survive.'

Hair is an integral part of the self for most in Western society, particularly for women. It is a sign of womanhood, identity, and their sexuality. One study in which 32 women with diffuse alopecia were interviewed found that seven of them had severe marital and sexual problems. Another study of 120 women with androgenetic alopecia found that the biggest problems were an inability to style their hair, dissatisfaction with appearance, concern about the hair loss continuing, and worry about others noticing their hair loss. There were also emotional problems, including self-consciousness, jealousy, embarrassment, and feeling powerless to stop their hair loss. Most of these women were experiencing hair thinning – they did not have the more serious alopecia totalis or universalis.

What are the problems for men?

Balding may not be as big an issue for men as it is for women. That is not to say that alopecia totalis or universalis is not devastating – it is – but many men expect to go bald as they age, and in Western society they are also free to shave their heads and not look ridiculous.

Alopecia is very different from normal balding, which is acceptable in society. However, losing your hair in big patches, or becoming entirely bald, including eyebrows, eyelashes and beard, perhaps your entire body hair, is considered not to be. For some men, the loss of hair in alopecia is as serious as it is for most women, and the experiences of men should not be undervalued. It is not acceptable to say to someone with alopecia, 'Why not shave off what's left? It's OK to have a shaven head.'

The appearance of alopecia is not the same as the appearance of normal balding, so we should not pretend that alopecia is less of a problem for men because they 'expect to go bald'. Men have similar problems to women regarding such matters as identity and coping – the difference being that it is more acceptable in society for men to have no hair. We must remember, though, that going without hair by choice is not the same as going without hair because you have to.

8

Coping with alopecia

What we have found so far

There are various ways of dealing with alopecia, including developing your own methods of coping, dealing with family and friends (social issues will be dealt with in Chapter 9), and using practical aids such as wigs and tattoos.

Usually the most severe psychological problems are going to be faced by those with the more serious forms of alopecia, but that is not always the case. Many people who have lost small patches of hair can become deeply distressed by it.

If you have alopecia, you can at first feel distressed and utterly helpless. It can be difficult to draw on your own strengths, the ways you normally cope with stressful events. Your world has been turned upside down. You cannot turn to family and friends because you feel they are rejecting you (sometimes they *are* rejecting you, but mostly this is not the case). You might not be able to go to work for fear of ridicule. In all walks of your life you are met with dead ends, and it is difficult to make any progress.

Practical exercise

Take a blank piece of paper and make two columns. On one side write all the positive things that have occurred as a result of your alopecia. On the other, write all the negative things. Do not worry about being trivial – everything counts (including not needing to buy shampoo!). Once you have done that, work through the positive side and think about why each is a positive thing, and how they became positive. Then work through the negative side and think of a reason why they are negative. Once you have done this, think about ways in which you can make the negative more positive, so that you can learn to come to terms with the alopecia. Who might help you work out ways of making the negative things positive? Family? Friends? Do you believe you need professional help?

For instance, you might think that 'understanding myself better' is a positive thing. Why do you feel that you understand yourself better? This might be because you have had to sit down quietly and think things through, analyse your life in a way that you never did before because you were too busy. Christopher Reeves, the actor, recently said that since his accident, which left him paralysed from the neck down, he has spent a lot more time thinking. Before the accident he would be constantly on the move, not stopping to think. Now he has no choice. You are led on then to the thought that perhaps alopecia is not as bad as being paralysed from the neck down. And it isn't!

On the other side of the list perhaps you put 'cannot go out in public'. That is a terrible thing, particularly if you were very gregarious, or if your work involves being in public. You have to find a way around that, and there are several practical things you might want to do.

Neil

'When I lost my hair I was teaching. The idea of going in front of a class, facing a group of students, with no hair, was a very difficult one for me. The first time I had to do it I asked the head of department to tell the students about my situation before I saw them. I asked her to tell the students that I had alopecia – not the background to why. I managed the class fine – after a short while it did not seem to matter. I was only self-conscious for the first few minutes. I look back now and think "Why did I need the students to know about my alopecia? It would have been pretty obvious at a glance!" The other difficult situation I had was when I was asked to be the usher at a friend's wedding. This was a friend I had not seen since I had lost my hair, and I knew many other friends would be there as well, other people I had not seen. I could not face taking a public role, meeting so many friends, with no hair, for the first time. I declined, explaining why I could not face the role. The friend was of course very supportive – that is what friends are!'

The case of Neil shows that friends can support you when you need support, and that is why they are friends. It may not help much reading this if you are in the throes of sudden hair loss, because you despair of receiving any support. You just feel that everyone will laugh. In reality, your real friends will not laugh.

It does not matter *how* you deal with social and work situations. What matters is that it works for you. There are several things you can do: wear a hat, wear a wig, wear a scarf, tell everyone beforehand what the problem is so that they do not look surprised when they see you (that can be painful). Discuss the problem over the telephone with them. Send people pictures of yourself. If it is a work situation, then possibly you are taking time off work. Explain the situation to your boss. Ensure you have medical support for your absence from work; you should speak to human resources, occupational health (if you have such a department), and perhaps your union if there could be problems. Most workplaces will be supportive. You do the job because you are good at it, and the boss and your colleagues will want you back. They will do their best to help you return.

When you are in the midst of despair it is good to remind yourself that you will receive support and sympathy from friends and work colleagues alike. They will not reject you; they will not shun you.

Stress, appraisal and coping

Dealing with stressful situations always involves an interaction between the stressful situation, an individual's appraisal of that situation, and their coping skills. This is about you learning to change what you can and manage what you cannot change. This does not just relate to hair loss (which you cannot change), but also to aspects of your life where you feel under stress. This might be at work, in your relationships, driving in heavy traffic, not having enough holidays. It might be what psychologists call 'daily hassles': those things that do not cause intense distress, but just bother you – such as your partner biting their nails, or trying to find something to eat for breakfast when it is dark and you want to be in bed, or being unable to find your clothes (you can no doubt think of many more reasons!). The point is, you have to learn to deal with these things by either changing them or managing them.

How to develop your coping skills

This section is about helping you to know what to do to help yourself, to make you stop feeling so awful. There is a whole range of coping styles that people use to help themselves. We are all different, so it is not appropriate to say which are going to be most effective for you. That is your decision.

Coping is related to personality, and we all have favoured ways of coping with problems. Some of us tend to avoid the problem as much as possible, others try to work out what has gone wrong and then resolve the difficulty. We can all develop our coping skills. Whatever your preferred method of coping, think about the suggestions below and try to incorporate them into your repertoire. It will help.

Psychologists have studied coping in some depth. There are a number of processes a person goes through when dealing with stress or illness. These include: working out the problem, adaptation, and coping itself. These processes do not occur in isolation – we move backwards and forwards through the stages. We will deal with each process in turn.

1 Working out the problem

Alopecia creates disequilibrium – our notions of selfhood, persona and identity have all been damaged, often irreparably. But the first thing we need to do psychologically is to appraise the situation. What does having alopecia mean to me? How is it going to affect my life? How am I going to deal with it? We need to draw on our knowledge and understanding – which tends to be very little in most people. Very few of us know anything about alopecia before we get the disorder – though most of us soon know a lot about it! We can also draw on the support of others.

2 Adaptation

There are a number of ways in which we can learn to adapt to alopecia. Two psychologists, Moos and Schaefer, when talking about adapting to illness in general, have proposed seven tasks. These can be separated into illness-related tasks and general tasks:

Illness-related tasks

- *Dealing with the symptoms*. In this instance it is loss of hair, and possibly related disorders such as eczema, asthma and problems with fingernails. Psychological distress, anxiety and depression are also symptoms.
- *Dealing with treatment*. This is likely to be difficult for you, as

69

treatments can be costly, lengthy, painful – and perhaps ineffective. It also involves making choices about whether to accept treatment or not, and which types of treatment to try.

• *Developing relationships with health professionals.* This may involve your GP, dermatologists, therapists, and perhaps alternative/ complementary therapists.

General tasks

• *Preserving an emotional balance.* You must try to compensate for the negative emotions (distress, sadness, anger) experienced by drawing on positive emotions (happiness, joy, love).

• *Preserving self-image, competence and mastery.* This has been dealt with in detail in Chapter 4. For many people with alopecia this will involve dealing with disfigurement and coming to terms with an altered identity.

• *Sustaining relationships with family and friends.* It is important for you to maintain social support networks, and this can be problematic if you feel that other people are mocking or ostracizing you. Family and friends will not be mocking you. They will want to support you – though they may not know how.

• *Preparing for an uncertain future.* Alopecia involves loss, and for some people this is permanent loss. If this is the case, then it is important for you to come to terms with the loss and redefine the future.

3 Coping styles

There are a number of ways in which people cope with difficult situations, and it might be useful for you to examine your own coping styles. The following questionnaire will help you to do this. Once you have worked out which coping strategies you use most effectively, you might like to think about how you can apply these to best effect when dealing with your alopecia.

THE ALOPECIA COPING SCALE

Please complete the following with reference to how you deal with your alopecia. Indicate on a 1–4 scale how often you use the coping style.

1 = strongly disagree
2 = disagree
3 = agree
4 = strongly agree

1 Active processing and planning

1 I like to actively cope with the feelings associated with my alopecia by thinking them through carefully.____

2 I tend to think about what the problem is relating to my alopecia before I act.____

3 I tend to try and solve my problems concerning alopecia rationally rather than emotionally.____

2 Focused attention

4 When a problem arises because of my alopecia I tend to focus on it before everything else.____

5 I like to clear my mind of other things in order to try and solve the problem.____

6 I am good at concentrating on solving problems arising because of my alopecia.____

3 Social support

7 I rely on my friends and family to help me.____

8 I cannot cope well with my alopecia if my family and friends aren't there to help.____

9 It is good to talk about my alopecia with loved ones.____

4 Positive growth

10 Stressful situations such as having alopecia help develop a mature mind.____

11 Good always comes out of a difficult situation such as alopecia.____

12 I know that in the end I will be a better person because of my alopecia.____

71

5 *Acceptance*
13 I have learned to live with my alopecia.____
14 Alopecia has happened. I can deal with it.____
15 I accept myself as I am now with alopecia.____

6 *Religion*
16 I know that my god has a reason for giving me alopecia. ____
17 God will help me deal with alopecia.____
18 God will help me come to terms with the stress caused by my alopecia.____

7 *Letting emotions out*
19 When my alopecia makes me sad, I freely cry.____
20 I am good at expressing my emotions with friends and family.____
21 I can express my positive emotions as well as my negative emotions about alopecia.____

8 *Denial and avoidance*
22 I refuse to accept my alopecia.____
23 I avoid thinking about my alopecia.____
24 I use alcohol or other drugs to stop me thinking about alopecia.____

9 *Drugs*
25 Alopecia has made me drink more alcohol.____
26 Alopecia has made me use more recreational drugs.____
27 I smoke more now I have alopecia.____

10 *Lack of control*
28 I cannot control my life now I have alopecia.____
29 Alopecia has taken over my life.____
30 I do not have any control over my social or work life now I have alopecia.____

Now add up your score for each of the 10 coping styles, and then fill in Table 2. Your coping style is determined by your scores in each category. A high score is 10 or more, medium 6–9, and low, 5 or lower.

Coping style	Score	High/medium/low
1 Active processing and planning		
2 Focused attention		
3 Social support		
4 Positive growth		
5 Acceptance		
6 Religion		
7 Letting emotions out		
8 Denial and avoidance		
9 Drugs		
10 Lack of control		

Table 2   Scores for each of the 10 coping styles.

Interpretation of the results

You will see that some of the coping styles are positive, and some are more negative. The positive ones include: active processing and planning, focused attention, social support, positive growth, acceptance, religion, and letting emotions out. The negative categories are: denial and avoidance, drugs and lack of control. The more positive coping styles you use the better. If you score low on any of the positive styles, then you should consider whether you can start using it more. If you score high on any of the negative styles, then you should consider whether you should use that style less.

Of course, it is not as simple as that. The negative styles are sometimes positive. For example, there is nothing wrong with going out for a drink (or even several) to forget once in a while, but it becomes a problem when you do it regularly or to excess. Similarly, for those of you who do not believe in a god, then religion is not necessarily a positive coping style – it is entirely neutral! You should examine your pattern of coping styles and see whether you should think about trying to change it.

But what do the different coping styles mean?

1 Active processing and planning

This is used by people who like to think through what the problems are relating to the stressful situation. If you stop and think why you are experiencing particular emotions and try to think of ways of resolving any problems, or if you think about how your alopecia affects you and then devise ways to stop it affecting you badly, then you are an active processor and planner.

2 Focused attention

This is a very useful coping style. Many people cannot deal with their problems because they won't focus on them, think about them, or try to find ways of dealing with them.

3 Social support

Social support is very important to people with alopecia. Many of us rely on family and/or friends to help us come to terms with our problems. We can often think through what is troubling us better if there is someone there as a sounding board, and we are better able to cope if there is someone to give us a hug when we are down.

4 Positive growth

This is perhaps the most positive coping style! Those of us who can think ahead to realize that good can come out of stressful situations often deal with everyday problems more effectively. Stressful situations are good for us. They help us understand the meaning of life – and that is not a trivial statement.

5 Acceptance

In the end, if the problem cannot be resolved, then we either have to learn to live with it, or learn to live with the continual stress and negative emotions associated with the problem. This is very true for people with permanent alopecia.

6 Religion

This is self-explanatory. Many people rely on God or religion to help them deal with stressful situations, and prayer and meditation can help quieten an unsettled mind.

7 Letting emotions out

Some people store up their emotions, unable to let go and have a good cry, believing that expressing emotions is a weakness. The reality is that, for many of us, being able to express emotions openly can help us deal with difficult situations.

8 Denial and avoidance

Many people refuse to recognize there is a problem – and one difficulty for psychologists is knowing whether a person is refusing to accept there is a problem, or whether they really do feel fine! Just because someone is not showing distress does not mean they are in denial. On the other hand, refusing to accept a problem can be psychologically damaging.

9 Drugs

Many people turn to drugs as a means of coping – and as a means of forgetting. There is nothing wrong with the occasional use of, for example, alcohol, for exactly that purpose. The problem arises if you are regularly using drugs for that purpose. Doctors can provide help for people who have drug problems.

10 Lack of control

This is very difficult for many people with alopecia, as the condition takes control away from you. You have no control over your hair, you feel you have no control over your appearance, even your identity has changed. This need not be the case, though – you can take back control of your life.

We use different coping strategies in different situations. As we said above, drinking alcohol is not a good coping style, though there are occasions when it is perfectly acceptable to have a few drinks (if you are already a drinker) and forget about your alopecia for a while. Be careful, though, for it might make you more depressed. The point is, every coping strategy may be appropriate on occasion, but some coping strategies are more positive and will help you progress more than others. Remember – there is no right answer, only what is right for you.

Coping questionnaires and scores do not provide answers on how to cope. They are simply a means of helping us to discover something about ourselves – assuming we have completed them honestly! In reality, we all use most of the above coping styles, partly depending on the situation, and partly depending on our own personalities.

Appraisal-focused coping

This kind of coping involves logical analysis and mental preparation for dealing with alopecia, turning what appears to be an unmanageable situation into a manageable one. It involves cognitively redefining the situation, accepting that the alopecia is real, and that it may be permanent, and redefining the situation in a positive way that is acceptable to you. Appraisal-focused coping may also involve cognitive avoidance and denial, attempting to minimize the seriousness of the situation. This is not going to be easy, but in the end it can be very successful.

Problem-focused coping

This involves confronting the alopecia and reconstructing your thoughts to make it manageable. There are three types of problem-focused skills.

In the first place you are likely to seek information and knowledge. Most of us have very little knowledge or awareness of alopecia, for it is not something widely discussed in society. Therefore it is normal that when you get alopecia, you try to find out as much as you can about it (like getting hold of this book!).

The second part of problem-focused coping involves taking action, learning specific procedures relating to treatment, learning about the chances of recovery, what is the likely time course of the alopecia, etc.

The third stage involves identifying alternative rewards – the developing and planning of events and goals that provide short-term satisfaction.

Emotion-focused coping

This involves managing emotions and maintaining your emotional equilibrium. Emotion-focused coping involves efforts to maintain hope when dealing with the stressful situation; it also involves what can be termed 'emotional discharge' – venting our feelings of anger or despair. Eventually, for people who are not going to have hair regrowth, there must be resigned acceptance, which involves coming to terms with the hair loss.

Individual factors

Of course, not everyone will respond in the same way to alopecia, and psychologists suggest that there are three factors that will determine the pattern of coping. These include:

1 Demographic and personal factors such as age, sex and socio-economic status.
2 Physical, social and environmental factors such as social support networks and the acceptance of one's physical environment.
3 Alopecia-related factors such as the disfigurement or stigma.

You will need to try to deal with the crisis caused by the alopecia via the stages of appraisal, the use of adaptive tasks, and coping skills. The particular pattern of tasks used may determine the psychological outcome of experiencing alopecia, in terms of quality of life. It is important to make effective use of coping in order to manage life.

Different coping strategies may be relevant at different times. Problem-focused coping may be particularly relevant in the early stages – learning to deal with having no hair in public situations, coping with the cold, etc. Later on, emotion-focused coping styles may be more important, when you are learning to come to terms with relationships or identity change, etc.

Crisis theory suggests that people are motivated to re-establish a state of equilibrium and normality. Alopecia leads to disequilibrium, so it is natural that you will need to re-establish a balanced sense of self. Psychologists suggest that we all have a search for meaning, a search for mastery, and a process of self-enhancement. These processes can be damaged when you first get alopecia; but they will quickly become re-established in most of us. Unfortunately, in some people there is a maladaptive response that makes it difficult to cope.

Keith

Keith experienced alopecia shortly after the death of his father. He was having difficulty dealing with the loss, particularly as his father had died quite young. Keith lost most of the hair from his head. Medical treatments were not successful, so he quickly gave them up. Over a period of several months some of his hair grew back, but whenever something stressful happened, either at home or at work, it dropped out again. To begin with, Keith did not have the personal resources to cope properly. He was depressed about his father, and was traumatized by the alopecia. He would sit at home, refusing to go out and see his friends, preferring to forget about everything, and watch television all night. He allowed his social support network to disintegrate, and thought he was ugly now that he had alopecia.

Fortunately, Keith had a close friend, James, who would not give up on him. James persisted in going to see Keith, though he usually got a poor reception. Then one day Keith realized what was happening. He was losing his friends; he was performing poorly at work. He was very unhappy, and made a decision to change. He telephoned James, who came round, and they sat up all night talking. Keith had moved from denial and avoidance towards an acceptance of his alopecia and a decision to actively do something about it. From then on, he slowly re-established his support networks, and became happier. 'I realized that life must go on, that my father was dead, that I had lost my hair – but it wasn't the end of the world. I still had my friends, my job, and my family. Fortunately, they waited for me.'

Jane
Jane worked in advertising. It was a stressful job, with tight deadlines and stroppy clients. When she discovered patches of hair loss, she realized that she had alopecia. She saw her GP who suggested it might be caused by stress. Over a single weekend, she worked out that it must be caused by her work – nothing else in her life was stressful – and made the decision to change her job for a much less stressful one. She managed to find a position working in the personnel department of a public company and was much happier. It was then that her hair started to grow back.

Psychological help

Psychologists have developed a range of techniques to deal with more serious forms of psychological problems. The techniques are used in therapy for depression and anxiety-related disorders, and many other types of problem.

The most effective techniques that may be applied to someone with alopecia are cognitive and behavioural strategies. It is not suggested here that you treat yourself formally, or that your problems are such that a clinical psychologist must deal with them, but that you yourself can apply the techniques that we are going to describe.

Caveat

If you have serious psychological problems as a result of your alopecia, please go and see your GP and explain the situation. There are various options your GP can use – he or she can prescribe medication for anxiety and depression which, while it may be effective at reducing the symptoms in the short term, will not resolve the problems caused by alopecia. Medication can be very useful in reducing your symptoms in order for you to function properly at work, with your family, or in your social life, but in the end the problems must be faced. Alternatively, your GP may refer you to a clinical psychologist or a psychiatrist, who will help you gain acceptance of your situation and help make appropriate changes to your life.

In this section, we will examine cognitive therapy and then behavioural therapy. When a person is being treated, these are not necessarily kept separate; an individual is treated according to need at the particular time, which will vary through the course of treatment.

Treatment with a clinical psychologist normally takes place over a period of several weeks or a few months. The patient, or client, is normally seen once a week for up to an hour. They are expected to do 'homework' between the sessions, which may involve keeping a diary, practising relaxation techniques, etc. The first session does not involve formal treatment; it is used for assessment. It is important for the clinical psychologist to carry out a thorough analysis or assessment of exactly what is wrong with the person. Treatment is always tailored to the specific needs of the individual based on this initial assessment, so this stage is very important.

At the end of treatment, the patient is assessed on various measures to ascertain the degree to which they have improved. Post-treatment follow-up is also used to ensure that improvement persists. Mental disorders are often not as simple as physical disorders; where they depend on the environment (as is the case with the response to alopecia), then there is the possibility of further problems arising post-treatment.

Psychological therapy is not always about cure, or about getting you back to how you were before the problem started, it is often about teaching you to deal with the disorder, to use better coping strategies, or to learn to relax, or have more rational beliefs about yourself.

Some medical practitioners do recognize that drugs are not the best way to treat alopecia, and that related stress can best be dealt with using psychological techniques such as relaxation, sometimes in conjunction with drugs. One study demonstrated this, showing that relieving stress has a favourable impact on the immune system.

What we are presenting here is not an alternative to treatment. It is a set of guidelines and ideas that you may find helpful. If you believe yourself to be seriously ill psychologically, then you should visit your GP for advice.

How stressed are you?

There are many questionnaires available to help you find out how stressed you are – try completing the following one. It will give you some idea not only of how stressed you are, but the ways in which you are stressed. Understanding what causes you problems is the first stage in finding ways to deal with these problems. The questionnaire examines the symptoms and problems precipitated by stress, stressors in your life, and your current coping styles. Symptoms of stress result not only from the stressors in your life, but the ways in which you appraise those stressors and how you cope with them.

First, though, it would be helpful to know in which areas you are experiencing problems.

Stress Questionnaire

Unlike many questionnaires, the following requires you to think of the problems you have, rather than provide you with a list to tick off. The effects of stress are very different for all of us. What is important for one person is irrelevant to the next. We would like you to spend some time thinking about each question, and provide

80

yourself with detailed responses where possible. It will help you come to terms with what causes you problems and the ways you deal with these.

When you are under stress, do you experience any of the following symptoms? Try to identify when and where you experience them.

1 *Physical symptoms?* For example: ulcers, high blood pressure, nausea, rapid heart rate, fatigue, dry mouth, headaches, sweaty palms, teeth grinding, hair falling out.

2 *Cognitive problems?* For example: difficulty in concentrating, worrying about hair loss, memory problems, problem-solving, reasoning, decision-making.

3 *Emotions?* For example: guilt, anger, anxiety, fear, panic, moodiness, hopelessness.

4 *Behavioural problems?* For example: sleeping problems, contact with others, relaxation, behaving inappropriately with others.

5 *Other problems?* For example: drinking or smoking to excess, loss of control of money, eating or drinking too much.

Which of the above problems are the most serious? List those you consider to be most problematic.

Which everyday situations ('daily hassles') cause you most problems? Examples include: arguing, children, preparing meals, travelling to work, financial difficulties, relationship problems, meeting deadlines, weight control.

What activities help you to reduce your stress? Examples might include walking, painting, running, reading.

Which of these do you find are best for reducing stress?

Are there any of these activities ones you feel you do not do enough?

Which of your stress-reducing activities work? Which symptoms do they not work for? How might you introduce ways of rectifying this?

Once you have detailed the ways in which you experience stress, you need to think about how you can learn to reduce or manage the stress. Dealing with alopecia is a particular problem, because the alopecia may not go away and you will have to learn to live with the disorder.

Stress management is not about getting rid of the stress you experience, but learning how to deal with it. There are a number of ways of dealing with stress, which we will now consider.

Cognitive therapy

Aaron Beck, who worked initially with people with depression, is perhaps the most famous name in cognitive therapy. He held the view that depressed people hold negative beliefs, which are conclusions based on faulty logic. A depressed person believes that they are humiliated or rejected, or that they are in some way deprived. The classic view put forward by Beck was that the depressed individual has a negative view of the self, a negative view of the world, and a negative view of the future. Depressed people, even when you give them evidence that contradicts their negative beliefs, will find some way of interpreting this badly. There is a negative bias in their reasoning.

The purpose of cognitive therapy is to rectify these false beliefs.

If you have alopecia, you can perhaps see how people with this condition might fit into this pattern of false beliefs. When your hair falls out, it is easy to start believing in the negative triad:

82

1 *I have a negative view of myself.* I look awful. I have no face left. I am unattractive. My hair was my most positive feature. Now I have nothing left. I am nothing. I am worthless.

2 *I have a negative view of the world.* I know that everyone is laughing at me. They think I look stupid/comical. I cannot go back to work. I cannot face my family. I cannot go to the pub for a drink. I cannot go to a restaurant. I cannot leave the house – even to go for a walk.

3 *I have a negative view of the future.* Now my hair has dropped out it will never grow back. I will never be attractive again. I will never be able to cope with life. Everyone will always hate me and laugh at me.

Identifying these negative beliefs forms the start of the therapy. Write down your own beliefs about having alopecia. Be honest, and be detailed. Do your beliefs fit into the triad set out above?

The next stage is to think about these beliefs, and determine whether they are rational, and then to try and alter the way you think about things. For instance, if you believe that you have a negative view of the world, that people are going to laugh at you if they see you walking down the street, have you considered why? Would you laugh at someone with alopecia? Of course not. At worst you might wonder what is wrong with them. The only time we really get exposed to such hair loss is in cancer treatment, so you might get people feeling sorry for you. Most people will simply treat you like they treat other people.

Will your friends laugh at you and ostracize you? Have you tested this belief? No. If you did, you would find that there is not a single friend who would laugh at someone in this predicament. You *can* go out with your friends and enjoy yourself.

This is not an easy task to do on your own. If you are depressed because of your alopecia, then it is unlikely that you are going to be able to deal with this difficult task all at once. Don't worry. Take your time. Make yourself think clearly. Write things down on pieces of paper. Think things through. If it helps, get one of your friends or a member of your family to talk it through. Just do not expect a family member to be a therapist. They are not. Also, you must remember that they may also be having problems coming to terms with your alopecia. You have to accept this. You have to become psychologically strong – and that can be very difficult.

Diary

Another technique you may find useful is to keep a diary. Fill it in with incidents that have occurred, and thoughts that have come to you during the day. This is a good way of having a conversation with yourself, of working your thoughts through. You can include elements about your beliefs, and also about the ways you are trying to change these beliefs. Write down the social situations you were in, how you dealt with them, how you felt, and how you might have dealt with them better. Review the diary once a week, marking off the points where you achieved something positive; noting the areas where you need to improve. When you have completed this for a few weeks, you will see if you are making progress. If you are, then congratulate yourself. Give yourself a treat. If not, review how you are dealing with your alopecia. What is blocking your progress?

Behavioural techniques

Behaviourism originated about a hundred years ago, when Pavlov trained his dogs to salivate at the sound of a bell. Since then, there has been a lot of research into behaviourism. Many psychologists have rejected it as a simplistic way of explaining human behaviour – but the reality is that it works, and so it is widely used by clinical psychologists. Perhaps we are not as complex as we think we are!

Clinical psychologists use a range of behavioural techniques in order to treat certain disorders. Behaviour therapy involves first learning to relax and then confronting the problem. It works on the idea that if we can learn to relax when we are in a situation that makes us anxious, then we will be better able to deal with that situation.

For instance, if you have alopecia and cannot face walking down the street with a bare head – the very thought makes your stomach turn – then if you learn relaxation techniques you can apply them as you walk down the street so it makes the situation bearable. Even before you walk down the street, go through the process of imagining yourself walking down it in a relaxed fashion. This is a general rule: imagine yourself in the stressful situation before you actually do it. Imagine yourself carrying out the activity while relaxed. You will find some specific relaxation techniques later in this chapter.

Behaviour therapy can be split into two fundamental types, flooding and systematic desensitization. They are used wherever someone feels anxious, particularly with phobias (having alopecia and refusing to go out in public is a kind of social phobia).

Flooding

This is where you are taught relaxation techniques and are then forced into the situation that makes you frightened. As your anxiety level rises you are reminded of the relaxation techniques and encouraged to use them. The theory here is that if you are put in the situation that makes you most anxious and are kept there, eventually your anxiety levels will reduce and you will be able to cope with the situation – you will realize that you do not need to be anxious.

This technique is always carried out under the supervision of a qualified psychologist – it is not something you should try yourself as it may be potentially harmful.

Systematic desensitization

This is a slightly less distressing form of dealing with anxiety-inducing situations. Again, you are first taught to relax, and the therapist will ask you to outline which situations make you anxious. You will probably be able to name a number of such situations; you will then be asked to rate each one, according to how anxious each would make you feel. The therapist then works from the least anxiety-provoking to the most anxiety-provoking situation, helping you to learn to relax at each one before moving on to the more serious situations. The theory here is that once you learn to stay relaxed in one context, it will be easier to learn to stay relaxed in the more difficult ones, so eventually you will be able to deal with those difficult situations.

For instance, you might list the alopecia-related anxiety-provoking situations to include: being seen without your wig in the house, going to the shops, public speaking, driving the car, going to the hairdressers (assuming you have alopecia areata), going to the dentist, and visiting friends and relatives. You might list visiting friends and being seen without the wig in the house as least anxiety-provoking, and public speaking as the most anxiety-provoking. Once you have put the incidents in order, from the least anxiety-provoking to the most, you can work on learning to be relaxed in the easiest first. Once you have mastered this you then move up the scale, event by event, until you learn to relax even with the worst situation.

The success of flooding and systematic desensitization is highly variable. It depends a lot on the strength of the patient to put up with the anxiety that will inevitably be induced. If the patient is very willing, then both techniques can be successful. The important point is that the patient must be ready for treatment.

You will see how both techniques can be applied to alopecia, but you first need to learn to relax.

Relaxation

Learning to sleep

Sleep problems can lead to excessive tiredness and irritability during the day, and eventual physical illness. There are a number of rules you can use to learn how to sleep more effectively:

- Set a specific time for going to bed and getting up. Have a lie-in at the weekend, but try to keep to the times during the week. Do not go to bed too early. One of the problems some people have is that because they are constantly tired they try going to bed early, and this can lead to waking in the night and problems going back to sleep again. Put the light on when the alarm goes off. This will counteract seasonal affective disorder (SAD). Try to relax your muscles when you get up.
- If possible, and if you want to, take an afternoon nap. The Spanish have the right idea. However, ensure that it is limited – 10–30 minutes depending on need and circumstance. Find a quiet place and relax; do not allow yourself any longer than your fixed time.
- Take regular exercise, but do not exercise immediately before going to bed.
- Keep the bedroom cool and ventilated. A warm airless room is not conducive to sleep.
- Have a bath before going to bed.
- Do not eat chocolate immediately before bed. Do not drink tea or coffee in the evening. All these contain caffeine, which is a stimulant, and will keep you awake. A rough rule is not to have any of these after 5 p.m. Have a glass of warm milk and honey instead.

- Some people prefer to read before sleeping, others need music, and others need a dark quiet room. Do what is appropriate for you.
- Think of something pleasant to help you drift off. No advice here, just use your imagination!

Meditation

Meditation is a special form of relaxation where you try to make your body calm. It is a series of mental exercises; there is evidence that meditation: improves mood, reduces intrusive and negative thoughts, secretes endorphins, increases the T-cell count, decreases the heart rate, and lowers blood pressure. Research has also shown that meditation can decrease anxiety, increase self-esteem, and lead to a more positive mood.

How to meditate

1 Incorporate meditation into your everyday schedule, a few minutes sometime in the day when you will not be disturbed. If possible, make it the afternoon, because that is when many of us become tense and tired. Do not take any stimulants before meditating, because they will keep your body aroused. Meditation should be a part of your healthy approach to exercise and nutrition, all of which contribute to reducing stress.
2 Select a quiet place to meditate.
3 Position yourself in a comfortable chair, in a comfortable position with your feet on the floor and your hands in your lap. Become passive, focus on a single object, on breathing, on a point in space. Do not let your mind wander; do not become distracted. If you are distracted by something unpleasant, bring yourself back by thinking of something pleasant, or simply focusing on your breathing.
4 Go through all your body with your mind to discover which areas are tense. Exercise any tense areas by gently moving the muscles of that area. Focus on your internal bodily processes, such as your heartbeat or your breathing.
5 Breath diaphragmatically, i.e. in through your nose; hold your breath for a brief period, and then breathe out through your mouth. Contract your abdomen.
6 Use a mantra, a calming phrase that you repeat while you are

meditating, such as 'relaxed body, clear mind', or 'I feel happy'. Do whatever feels right for you.

7 Use visualization. A prisoner of Stalin, incarcerated in the Gulag, mentally built a house, brick by brick, over the years he was imprisoned. You start by selecting the area you want to live, whether by the sea, on a hill, etc. Design the house, then prepare the ground, put in the foundations, gradually build it brick by brick, taking care to select the right type of windows and doors. Eventually you will be able to decorate and furnish the house.

8 If you wish, use relaxing music.

9 Do not rush. Some of you may be Type A personalities, who want everything NOW, and so if you try to relax too quickly you may become more tense. Slow it down!

10 After the meditation exercise, give your body a chance to readjust by stretching. Do not stand up too quickly or you might feel dizzy.

Do not try to do too much at once. Start with just five minutes, and try to build up over a period of time to 15 or 20 minutes. Meditation is a skill to be learned. What is right for one person may not be right for the next, so do not think you have to follow the above rules rigidly. The important thing is that it works for you.

Progressive relaxation

This is a technique proposed by Jacobsen. Every time a muscle contracts it creates a series of neural impulses that are sent to the brain. This leads to tension, particularly if a wide range of muscles are involved. The purpose of progressive muscular contraction is to enable people to recognize when excessive muscle contraction occurs, and how to relax these muscles to reduce the tension. It is a technique used by therapists, but you can apply the main principles yourself.

This is a widely used technique, which may be suitable for people who do not feel comfortable with meditation.

1 Practise at home without distractions.
2 Use a comfortable but firm mattress.
3 Practise before eating if possible.
4 Lie quietly for 3–4 minutes with your eyes closed.

5 Do not flex damaged muscles.
6 Bend your left hand upwards while your arm is supported on the bed. Observe the tenseness in the upper arm.
7 Release the hand, feel the change in tension.
8 Repeat the movement.
9 Repeat the exercise using the other joints of the upper body – elbows, shoulders, neck, head.
10 Repeat this with the joints of the lower body – ankles, knees, hips and buttocks. Then do the same with the abdominal muscles.
11 Flex the muscles of the face by changing your expression. Look to each side without moving your head and feel the tension in the eyeballs.

Do not hurry through the muscle groups – take your time. You must feel comfortable with what you are doing. You can use relaxing music if you wish. The more you practise, the better you will become at relaxing. If necessary, you can carry out the exercises while sitting in a chair, perhaps on a bus, plane or train. You should also think about your posture – how you sit and stand all day. Are there ways you can improve it? Do not slouch, do not stay in the same position for too long. If your work is a desk job, make sure you get up regularly and walk around.

Again, you should link these exercises to your daily routine of exercise and nutrition.

At the beginning you may not manage to carry out relaxation techniques for very long. This does not matter; take it slowly and build up the time. Perhaps start with five minutes, and gradually build up over a number of weeks. Remember, there is no right or wrong, and the aim of relaxation is for you to *relax*, so do not worry if you are distracted. Skills take time to develop.

There is evidence that relaxation can reduce blood pressure, change your brain waves, reduce intake of alcohol and cigarettes, and help change lifestyle. Other research suggests that relaxation is no better than normal resting; but if you are not very good at spontaneous resting, then relaxation should help!

Image therapy

This is a simple technique used after you have relaxed. Try to visualize the image that, 'the hair root cells become healthy by receiving nutrients from the rich blood flow where I have alopecia'. Then try 'all head hair grows', and 'I am very self-confident'. Throughout this, which should take up to 20 minutes, try to imagine your hair growing.

This is a technique that has been used with cancer patients. It is difficult to ascertain whether it is effective, and whom it might be effective for, but there is some evidence in its favour.

Nutrition

The advice here is simple: eat fresh food; have a balanced diet. Do not avoid any unhealthy foods that you enjoy – just eat them in moderation. Do not use artificial nutrients such as vitamin tablets, unless instructed to do so by your GP. Avoid heavily processed foods – junk foods – which are often high in fats and sugars, and low in vitamins and micro-nutrients that are essential to maintain health.

There are specific things that can aid hair growth. You should eat plenty of eggs and liver, which provide vitamin A; dark green leafy vegetables, carrots and sweet potatoes for beta carotene; vegetable oils, nuts and oily fish for essential fatty acids; and shellfish, red meat and pumpkin seeds for zinc.

You will get all you need from a healthy diet. Listen to your body – it will tell you which nutrients it needs.

Exercise

Nutrition and exercise are perhaps the two most important contributors to general good health. The type of exercise you do is less important than making sure you do the exercise regularly. If you have not exercised for years, do not try to do too much at once. There is little point in someone who has not been running for 20 years trying to start by running several miles. It will hurt, and you may suffer an injury. It is better to start with relatively light exercise and build up slowly. Exercise specialists recommend a minimum of 20 minutes' exercise, three times a week. Find something you enjoy and do it.

Giving meaning to the trauma of hair loss

For those of us for whom alopecia is, or has been, a traumatic experience we can try to think how alopecia has not just been something negative in life, but also something positive. There is truth to the statement that out of a traumatic experience we can grow psychologically, and life can take on extra meaning through the development of understanding.

Religion and spirituality

Many people turn to their gods in times of crisis. Such beliefs can be a very effective way of coming to terms with and understanding why you have got alopecia and how you can deal with it. It is not our purpose to describe the range of religions that offer support to individuals in times of crisis. If you have a religious belief, then you will know how you can obtain support, perhaps through praying, or visiting a priest.

For some, one of the purposes of a set of spiritual beliefs is to provide an explanation for the world and the events in it. If you hold such beliefs, then you may believe that there is a reason for your alopecia. This in itself can provide comfort – scaffolding on which to base your coping.

9

Relationships

Jake

'For me, the consequences of my alopecia universalis did not end with the hair loss, they had barely begun. I had only recently become a father, so perhaps there were more emotions around than usual. I do not know how far this might provide an explanation for what happened. From this distance (12 years), perhaps I am more forgiving than I was. My hair loss started almost the moment my best friend died. I remember it all very clearly. I found out about the death on the telephone on Remembrance Sunday. I was devastated, but there was worse to come. I was emotionally distraught, and under those circumstances we usually turn to our partners for a hug. I did. I didn't get one. I was turned away with, "You wouldn't be this upset if I died". My mind was suddenly emptied. I asked for a hug: "Even if you don't mean it, it will help me". I was turned away. I begged – literally. I was ignored. That was the end of our relationship, though we did not split up until more than three years later.

'That was the point my hair started to fall out.

'As my hair fell out of my head, as I lost my eyebrows, my eyelashes, I had lost my partner. Once my hair was gone she never looked me in the eyes again. She could not look at me. She couldn't stand the sight of me – and I mean that physically, not emotionally. It took me a long time to realize the relationship was dead – even after the rejection I did not accept it. I still tried to make things right. But it is very difficult when you have a partner, the mother of your baby, who won't even look you in the eye – because your eye doesn't look right. It was somebody else's eye. It was not mine.'

How can alopecia affect others?

Alopecia does not occur to someone in isolation. A friend or relative can be affected in two ways:

1 Responding to the emotions felt by the person with alopecia.

2 Responding to the physical changes brought about by the alopecia.

Both of these are real. Many people try to deny them – particularly the second – but something that has an impact on the identity of the person with alopecia may also affect how others perceive them. Identity is a social process; our perception of others is affected by how they look. People present themselves in a particular way in order that others perceive them in a particular way. So it is not surprising that when a fundamental change such as hair loss occurs, especially without warning, it can affect others.

Once this has been admitted, then the process of understanding and adapting to the alopecia can begin. Do not be afraid that you might initially have negative feelings regarding the way a person looks. *You* have to adapt, as well as the person with alopecia. However, it is not impossible. You have the relationship with them because of the person, not the fact that they have hair!

Depending on your own situation, you may be well aware of these social consequences. Many people with alopecia simply do not go out. They cannot face the world. They cannot stand the idea of people laughing at them in public. Of course, we have to reach an understanding that people in the street, in the pub, or at work are not going to laugh. Most people will probably not even notice. If they do notice, they are likely to be unconcerned. If they do stare, then there are strategies for dealing with them (look back, ask if there is a problem, ask if they've never seen anyone without hair before, etc.).

This chapter focuses on the potential impact on other people. No two cases are alike, so what we are providing is not a definitive 'this will happen'. It will depend on the people involved, your relationships with them, and individual characteristics.

Marriages and partnerships

Unfortunately alopecia is a major cause of relationship breakdown. If either the person with alopecia or their partner cannot cope with the alopecia, then there may be relationship problems, possibly the loss of the relationship altogether.

One survey has shown that up to 40 per cent of women with

alopecia have experienced problems with their marriage. It will be both that they have problems with identity and self-esteem, and that their husbands or partners cannot cope. It is important that everything possible is done to ameliorate this, and Chapter 10 will deal with these issues.

It is important to note that many of these broken marriages may have been problematic before the alopecia began, and that the alopecia was simply the factor that finally ended the marriage. It is probable that some people get alopecia *because* of their unhappy marriages. These factors are difficult to tease out, but we must be clear that the reasons for the breakdown of a marriage are generally complex, and not just because one partner has alopecia.

Children

Children are a tricky subject, as the sight of a parent or sibling suddenly losing their hair can shock them. Older children will probably be aware of the effects of chemotherapy and may worry that their parent has got cancer and will die. Younger children will be confused and may become upset. They may think that their Mummy or Daddy has left them and has been replaced with a stranger – particularly if the alopecia occurs suddenly and is extensive. (This is a good example of how identity changes with alopecia – children do not have the social graces of adults, nor do they have the sophistication.)

It is important to tell children what is happening as soon as possible and in detail. They need to be told that alopecia is not a life-threatening disorder, and that it simply involves a change of appearance. It will be best in most circumstances if the transition for the children can be made easily and with limited emotion. Children are incredibly resilient and adaptable. Once they know what is happening, they will readily accept it. Sometimes they may lack social skills and say things like, 'I don't like your new hairstyle, Daddy. Can you grow it back again please?' Deal with this kind of thing positively. Say no, and explain why. Save your distress for when they are not around.

Other members of the family

Other members of the family, the people who do not live in the same house, may also have difficulties. They may have known you all your life. It is important that they receive information about the disorder, so that they are in a position to be supportive.

Friends

Friends will generally be great. You may not think so before you see them, but if we are talking about real friendship, then all you will receive is support and help. Friends are the people who often help you come to terms with your emotions. They are practical and helpful.

Social life

In the early stages of alopecia it is your social life that might be most affected, and this is because you do not want to be seen in public. There are various ways of dealing with this very stressful situation. The most difficult is to just go out and face the world. This is a form of 'flooding' (as mentioned earlier). Once you learn to venture out into the world you will realize that most people are simply not bothered what you look like. Strangers do not care at all, and friends get used to the change quickly. Again, it is a problem of personal perception as to what you *think* people think, and what they actually *do* think. Why not ask them?

If you need to, you can wear a wig or a hat in public, and then most people will not even notice that you have alopecia.

There is no reason whatsoever why you cannot have a normal social life. The only reason you have a problem is because of the way you think, not the way others think.

10

Helping someone with alopecia

This chapter is written to help those of you who have a member of your family, or a friend, with alopecia. It provides some guidance on how to help the person deal with the problem, and how you can help yourself deal with it. Alopecia does not just affect the person who loses their hair; it affects those around them too. Many family members and friends can also suffer emotionally as a result of the hair loss, and you have to know that this is acceptable and normal.

Talking

One of the most useful things to do when someone gets alopecia is to sit down and talk – seriously talk. Talk through all the issues that emerge. Talk together. If there are children, talk with them. Talk with parents. Talk with friends. Talk with your partner.

Talking will help. Everyone must have the chance to express themselves about how they feel regarding the alopecia. There is a time for thinking of the sufferers themselves, and there is a time for thinking about the people around them. If people are not allowed to talk they may start thinking about something and it may grow to trouble them. It may concern information; it may concern feelings. Throughout the book so far we have largely talked of the feelings and beliefs of the person with alopecia, to the detriment of those around them. True, it is worse for the person with alopecia, but there must be a recognition of the problems and issues facing their loved ones too.

A *caveat*

Talking about emotional problems is usually very difficult, and discussing emotional problems relating to alopecia with a partner can, depending on the circumstances of the partnership, damage the relationship. Two people who are very close are likely to be able to help each other by talking, but two people whose relationship is already lacking security, or is weak for whatever reason, may not survive alopecia. It is unlikely that people in a weak relationship will attempt what is discussed in this chapter, but it is important for everyone to be aware of the potential dangers.

If you believe your problems are very serious, go to your GP and ask to see a counsellor or a clinical psychologist. If your doctor believes your problems are particularly serious, he or she may prescribe appropriate medication, and then refer you to a therapist.

Alternatively, there are organizations such as Relate that offer help. If you are religious, you may wish to visit your spiritual adviser.

Social support

Social support works differently in men and women; one Japanese study showed that successful social support for men depends at least partly on the way they were brought up, while with women it depends more on personality. Successful social support for women is related to being extraverted and not neurotic. What is particularly interesting is that social support is not something that can be provided (or not provided) by the people surrounding someone with a problem, but is more related to the characteristics of the person. Their personality or background experience determines, at least in part, how successfully they can use social support.

This fits with our commonsense view of people. We all know people who depend a lot on social support and others who do not. That does not determine whether or not they experience stress-related problems or illnesses. It is an example of how we need to be aware of the needs of the person we are trying to help. We need to know not only when they need such support, but when they do not.

Helping skills

We are not proposing that you suddenly become a trained counsellor or a psychologist, but that you read this section, think about the issues, the skills involved, and consider how they could help you in your relationship, and how you might be able to support the person with alopecia by employing these skills.

You will not be able to act as a counsellor or therapist. Not only

are you not trained, but it is very difficult for even trained people to act as counsellors with their own family and friends. It is not appropriate. We all share emotional baggage.

Helping skills are not a set of skills that are out of the reach of the ordinary person; they are not something you need a degree to understand. They are what we use regularly in our everyday life. You, the individual who is dealing with someone who has alopecia, will know when that person is having problems. You are best placed to help them.

It is important to state from the outset that there are things that you probably should not do when you are taking on this role. These include:

- Trying to cheer the person up – this can make things worse. You need to know when you should be trying to cheer them up and when you should be providing support.
- Talking about yourself. Many of us do this, and it rarely helps.
- Trying to provide a solution to whatever is bothering the person. It is not that easy. Do not try and give advice at the wrong time.
- Thinking that being active, doing something, is important. There will be many occasions when just being there and responding to the person's wishes is all that is required.

Counselling has been around for as long as people have been, and some people are naturally good at helping others. They are good at sitting and listening, and helping people to resolve their own problems. It comes naturally to some of us, but the rest of us can learn. We have all counselled and been counsellors, so nothing here should be particularly surprising. We use these skills in any situation where people are having problems and their lives are being affected.

Why do you want to use these skills?

You want to use these skills to help the person with alopecia to manage their problems. Having this condition is difficult, and the more support someone with alopecia has the better. You are not there to provide solutions, but to be someone who supports others in finding their own solutions, helping them to live more happily, to learn to cope with their alopecia. It is about managing problems, not solving them. It is about enabling a person to draw on their own inner resources to sort out their problems.

The skills described here will help you when you are trying to deal with someone who has alopecia but is not coping well. You may find it useful to read the previous chapter too, as that contains some useful information about helping people to deal with alopecia.

Specific skills

There is a range of relevant skills, and you may already have some of these. You will be able to work on developing others. Do not expect to achieve them all to a high degree – you are not a professional. The skills are there to guide you in your interactions with the person with alopecia.

Empathy

Empathy is critical, as there has to be a capacity for understanding what the person is going through. This can sometimes be difficult. Some people seem to be naturally empathic, others are not. Not everyone can become empathic – it is a trait very few people can switch on and off at will (though we do know one clinical psychologist who has this ability – and it is probably a good coping strategy as a therapist).

Suspending judgement

You also have to suspend your judgement. This can be difficult for anyone, but if you are the husband, wife, parent, etc. of someone with alopecia it can be exceptionally hard. You feel you know what is good for them. But remember, you do not. Trying to advise someone who is experiencing emotional torture because of their alopecia how to think will be a disaster. Let them say what they want to say in the way they want to say it. Let them be the judge of their own emotions and feelings.

You want the person with alopecia to know that you have understood them. That will enable them to move on to the next phase.

Listening skills

When trying to help someone it is important to listen to them, and to listen carefully. Therefore listening is a communication skill, perhaps the most important such skill. But it is not just about listening to someone; it is also about talking. It is important to speak in order to clarify in your own mind what is being said, to obtain detail, to sort out ambiguities. Listening is an active skill, and the purpose of active listening is to allow the person to talk, to articulate the problem. Remember that the person with alopecia will not have an instant solution in their head; if they are emotionally disturbed (and why shouldn't they be?), then their thinking and feeling is going to be confused and fragmented. Active listening involves drawing out their story.

Listening does not come naturally to most people. Many of us do not listen to the other person when we are having a conversation. We know what we want to say before the other person has finished – if you want a good example of this, listen to politicians! Listening is a very difficult skill, but it is probably the most important one to learn if you want to help someone with alopecia.

You could start by *being listened to*. That is also difficult. Sometimes we have things to say that we think will sound silly to someone hearing them, particularly if we are confused about that person. But being listened to will help provide insight into the difficulties the person with alopecia may have in speaking to anybody about their problems.

When you are listening you will need to respond to the person speaking. These responses can take a number of forms:

1 *A probing response*. But be careful here. You are trying to get the person to talk, not to respond to questions. Use this technique to gather information that you feel the person is not providing spontaneously.
2 *An interpretative response*. Again, you need to take care not to over-interpret what the person is saying. That is their task. It is all too easy to try to put meaning on what a person says – it is a natural response that must be resisted.
3 *An evaluative response*. This is a moral question, and you should try to avoid pointing out whether the person is right or wrong. Again, that is their task. There is no right or wrong way to respond to alopecia. You are not there to have a debate.
4 *A supportive response*. Again, it is very easy to respond in a supportive manner, but you need to try and remain non-committal. This is going to be very difficult if you are close to the person, and it may not be possible. The person does not need advice and

sympathy, not when they are working through their problems. Advice and sympathy come outside the counselling role.

Being non-confrontational

It is important not to challenge what the person is saying. Do not allow yourself to criticize or put an opposing point of view. If the person is arguing irrationally, it is very likely they will pick it up themselves in the end. It is important that these decisions are made by the speaker, not the listener.

Showing acceptance

The person with alopecia is the one who must accept that they are stuck with negative beliefs or emotions. It is not for you to point that out.

Respect

Carl Rogers, an eminent therapist, said that respect involves liking and regard. His famous phrase involves 'unconditional positive regard'. This is very important if you are going to help someone close to you deal with their problems relating to alopecia. 'Unconditional' means that it does not matter what the person says; 'positive' means that you will continue to think well of them; 'regard' means that you will carry on respecting them.

If you are close to the person with alopecia it is likely that you respect them. Respect also involves having an open mind, accepting what the person says. Respect is a key part of any relationship, and any help that you – as a lay counsellor – can provide is likely to depend enormously on the respect you show the person with alopecia, and the beliefs and feelings they display. It is probably more important than anything else. If the person knows you respect them, even when they have opened up their deepest feelings, then the battle is half won. This particularly applies in alopecia, because one of the strongest feelings a person with alopecia might have is that no one will respect them – no one will treat them like a person any more.

Respect must involve the assumption that whatever the person says you will treat it with dignity and consideration, that their views are worth listening to.

Confidentiality

This is very important when using counselling skills. What the person says should be treated in confidence and not disclosed to others without the person's permission, and that should include other family members, however much you feel it may ultimately benefit the sufferer. The basic rule is, 'Don't gossip.'

Losing your own point of view

One of the reasons we do not tend to listen to people is that if we genuinely hear what the other person is saying and do not move on to provide our own point of view, then our point of view may be lost. When we are listening with respect, we are in danger of losing our own point of view.

The problem with alopecia is that it does not just hurt the person with alopecia; it hurts others too. If you are trying to support the person with alopecia and you are close to them, then losing your point of view is a very important issue. Under normal circumstances, if we talk to people in public (bar staff, taxi drivers, etc.), they tend to agree with us, just to ensure the social fabric is not undermined. When we argue, we argue in agreed circumstances, whether it is the classroom or the pub. In neither case do we lose our point of view.

If we *do* lose our point of view, the person we are trying to help will trust us and continue talking. However, this issue is made far more complex when we are being amateur counsellors – that is, helping a friend or partner with alopecia when that person is aware of our opinions. But that does not negate the value of using helping skills. This is not a formal counselling relationship. These skills are presented to help you support the person with alopecia work through their problems. But it may be that you, the one helping the person with alopecia, also needs help, whether informal or formal. Do not ignore your own needs.

Being genuine

This is something that should be relatively easy when you are helping someone with alopecia. It is likely, given that you already have a relationship with the person, that you are going to be genuine in your responses. Genuineness relates to your personality; it is concerned with sincerity.

Being tolerant

You are not perfect, but tolerance is important when dealing with someone with alopecia. If you are playing the role well, all their anger, fear and bitterness concerning their hair loss is likely to come out at some stage – and you must tolerate it.

Being hardworking

This is very important, and to succeed in helping the person with alopecia will require a lot of hard work from you. It will not be an easy task, and will be made all the harder because you may have your own issues to deal with regarding the alopecia.

Stages of helping

We are including this to give you an idea of how people are helped in a counselling situation.

Any helping situation passes through three stages:

1 The helper needs to understand the problem, which means that the other person has to define the problem in detail.
2 The helper should challenge the other person's ideas about the problem, which leads to them having to redefine the problem.
3 The helper should raise issues about the other person's resources, which should lead to them managing the problem better.

These three stages are not entirely independent, and there will be some overlap between them. You will see that there are similarities with the work of the clinical psychologist, discussed in the last chapter. Again we have the situation of trying to identify what the problem is, to get the person with alopecia to talk about it in detail. Only then can the search for a solution be started.

You are not necessarily going to try to work through these stages as a counsellor to the person with alopecia. If you *both* read this section, then you will see the need to progress through these stages, and you can help each other with the task. The skills of the previous section will be important throughout.

Stage 1: Understanding

The aim of this stage is for the person to be clear that the helper has fully understood their position, and that the person being helped is aware that they are stuck in a problem. There are a number of activities involved here, which involve applying the above techniques. The helper must pay attention, and encourage the person to present the whole story, to allow them to make sense of what is troubling them.

By the end of this phase it is important that the helper has understood the person's situation from the person's viewpoint. It is only then that progress to Stage 2 can take place.

Stage 2: Redefining the problem

Eventually the person with the problem will simply be repeating the same information and no progress will be made. It is important at this point to move on. Do not try to get into this stage too quickly – nor too slowly. Helping someone through a problem can be a difficult task!

It is at this point that we want the person with alopecia to make progress in the way they are thinking about the problem, to change the picture. Stage 2 really involves challenging the person's perspective, making them think about change. You need to probe more, draw them out.

This phase can be tricky because the helper has to encourage the person to change their perspective. This is difficult because the person with alopecia should be the one to make the change. It has to come from inside them, not from a helper.

Stage 3: Managing the problem

Stage 3 is about managing the problem: sorting out what options are available and choosing between them. Again, it is important that the person with the problem does the sorting out. This stage has a number of things to cover:

- *Creating the options.* There are probably quite a few of these, most of which the person with alopecia would not be aware of at the outset of the process. What are the options when going out in public with alopecia? These could include: a bare head, a hat, a scarf, a wig, or not going out at all.
- *Choosing between the options.* What is the best course of action? Some options are probably entirely impractical and should be discarded immediately; others need more careful consideration. With the options listed above, 'not going out at all' is probably not a sensible solution. We all need to go out shopping, eating and drinking, walking, or whatever. So the next thing is to decide between the more sensible options of going out without any head

covering, using a hat or scarf (sensible in winter!), or wearing a wig.

- *Putting the options into action.* It might be that different options suit different occasions. If the person with alopecia chooses to go out bareheaded, yet feels too anxious to do so, then it is time to do something about it. The last chapter described behaviour therapy, and how it is used to reduce anxiety. That is one course of action. Another might be to buy a wig for special occasions – going to the restaurant, for instance, as that might require a lot of self-confidence.

- *Measuring progress.* It may be important to monitor the success of the strategies used – for example, to explore whether the behavioural techniques have helped reduce the anxiety of walking down the street without any head covering, or whether a wig does give them self-confidence. If there are any problems with these stages, then back to the counselling skills. Work through the issues again.

How do you apply the three stages when you are not a counsellor?

The simple answer is that you do not – at least, not formally. The process remains the same though. In order for the person with alopecia to progress, to work towards resolving their problems, they have to be clear about what the situation is (Stage 1), think about ways of dealing with the issues (Stage 2) and deal with them (Stage 3). You can help with this process, not by being the formal counsellor, but by employing the skills appropriately.

However, the stages do not work as simply as described above. People do not work out what all their problems are, find ways of dealing with them, and only then actually deal with them. Instead they are more likely to move backwards and forwards between stages. New problems will arise and will be solved, then another problem will arise, and so on – until the person learns to deal with the alopecia.

Is this counselling?

No. We have described above the general process of counselling: the structure of the counselling programme, and the skills and methods used to enable you to help yourself. It is not for us to say how much of this you would wish to apply in your own situation. That will depend on circumstances, on your own skills; it will depend on your own feelings and emotions concerning the alopecia. What the above provides is a framework from which you can extract that which is most appropriate to your circumstances. We must reiterate that if there is a serious problem then you should approach a professional, who will be able to deal with the issues with a detachment that is rarely possible within a complex relationship.

11

Recovery from alopecia

What do we know?

We hope it will be clear by now that the time course and outcome of alopecia is far from predictable. However, there are certain things we (more or less) know:

- The more severe the alopecia, the lower the chances of regaining your hair.
- For most people, alopecia is patchy alopecia areata, for which there is a good chance of recovery – though there may be recurrences throughout life.
- Alopecia is an autoimmune disorder, caused by a combination of genes, personality and environmental factors.
- Alopecia is a disfigurement disorder, which can have serious consequences for identity.
- Alopecia is more common than we think; many people cover it up with a hat, a wig or a hairstyle.
- Medical treatments for alopecia have limited effectiveness.
- Some members of the medical establishment do not appear to understand that alopecia is a distressing condition.
- Some sufferers have difficulty coping and adapting to alopecia.
- Some people experience relationship difficulties.
- Many people successfully cope with, and adapt to having, alopecia.

There is still a lot of research to be carried out on alopecia. The biology of hair is fairly well understood, but exactly how alopecia occurs is not well understood. Once research has led to a greater understanding, then it is likely that genuine cures will start to be developed.

Alopecia is a disfigurement disorder, which has, as we have seen, major implications for identity and selfhood. Recovery from alopecia can be about rebuilding your 'self' and about rebuilding relationships anew, and this can take time. In the last few chapters

107

we have tried to show what the problems might be and how you can adapt to the changes involved. You *can* do this. You *can* recover. If you are in the early stages, or if your hair loss is still getting worse, or if you despair of ever being happy again, then just think to yourself it *will* get better. Individual differences play a very large part in recovery from alopecia. We cannot predict who will get their hair back; nor can we predict how people will learn to cope psychologically and socially.

We do hope that this book has provided some practical advice for those of you with alopecia. It is our view that understanding a disorder is the first stage in recovering from it, which is why we included all the work on immunology, stress, and how the hair cycle works. For something as potentially destructive as alopecia, it was important to include the chapters on the personal and social consequences of the condition, in order that you understand what is happening to you.

We also know there are tried and tested ways of recovering from a disorder, psychological techniques that can be applied to individual problems, and which can help you deal with the difficulties of that disorder, which is why we included the chapters on dealing with alopecia. In this chapter we wanted you to think of how you can develop positively through your experience of alopecia; how understanding yourself and your relationships can make you a more contented and fulfilled person.

Further information

There are a number of resources available to help you understand and deal with alopecia. One of the best places to start is your GP; he or she should be able to provide you with information and, if necessary, refer you to a dermatologist. If you are having emotional problems dealing with your alopecia, then your GP may refer you to a clinical psychologist or recommend a counsellor.

One of the best ways of understanding alopecia is to find out as much as you can yourself. As you will have seen, there has been quite a bit of research carried out in relation to the biology of alopecia, but relatively little regarding psychological issues. Most of this research is published in academic journals, and you may get advice from your local library or from the internet regarding accessing these journals.

Books

Inaba, M. and Inaba, Y., *Androgenetic Alopecia*, Springer-Verlag, 1996. At the time of writing (2003), this book was out of print. It provides detailed information about the hair cycle, challenging the three-phase theory, suggesting instead a four-phase cycle, involving stem cells. The main focus of the book is on male-pattern balding rather than alopecia areata.

Peterseil, Y. and Katz, A., *Princess Alopecia*, Pitpopany Press, 1999. This is a children's book about a person who develops alopecia, and is a useful read for children with alopecia. It examines many of the issues relevant to children.

Shapiro, J., *Principles of Diagnosis and Management of Hair Loss*, Martin Dunitz, 2002. This book is for specialist medical practitioners such as dermatologists, plastic surgeons, and GPs. It is concerned with the effective management of hair loss, though it is weak on psychological aspects.

Steel, E., *The Hair Loss Cure*, HarperCollins, 1999. This guide focuses on alopecia areata, baldness and thinning hair. It includes information on drug treatments, complementary treatment such as nutrition, aromatherapy, relaxation and meditation, and case histories. It is anecdotal rather than a systematic survey of the area, but it is still interesting to read.

Thompson, W. and Shapiro, J., *Alopecia Areata*, Johns Hopkins University Press, 1998. This text examines the various medical and alternative therapies, practical strategies for living with alopecia, and adjusting to living with a wig. The disadvantage for European readers is that it has an American focus.

Other books relate to dermatology and may mention alopecia. For instance:

Papadopoulos, L. and Bor, R., *Psychological Approaches to Dermatology*, BPS Books, 1999. This contains some information about alopecia, but is more general. Relevant areas are covered, such as body image, coping and counselling.

There are several books relating to hair loss and treatment, but these are not concerned specifically with alopecia.

Many books discuss the immune system, for example, Carlson, N. R., *Physiology of Behaviour*, 8th edition, Pearson, 2004.

Websites

http://www.keratin.com/
This is probably the most comprehensive site relating to hair. It has a lot of up-to-date information on alopecia, and also on other matters relating to hair.

http://www.ehrs.org/
The European Hair Research Society, an academic organization devoted to hair research in the widest sense.

http://npntserver.mcg.edu/html/alopecia/AlopeciaFAQ(part01).html
An extensive FAQ site; it is somewhat disorganized, but is interesting reading.

http://www.hairlineinternational.com/
Hairline International was set up by someone with alopecia in order to provide assistance to others.

*http://islandnet.com/~*sheila*/*
Sheila Jacobs's website. This has links to a wide range of alopecia-related material.

http://www.follicle.com/
General information on hair loss, including types of alopecia.

http://www.trichologists.org.uk/
Institute of Trichologists, a professional organization for people specializing in hair treatment.

http://www.bacp.co.uk/
The British Association for Counselling and Psychotherapy. This is a useful contact for finding out about counselling, and where to find a counsellor.

http://www.cfaces.demon.co.uk/
Changing Faces, an organization set up to help people, particularly children, deal with disfigurement.

http://www.alopeciaareata.com/
US National Alopecia Areata Foundation. This site contains a lot of information, focusing mainly on the USA.

Address

Children's Alopecia Society
PO Box 2505, 3 Uppertown Road, Eastbourne, East Sussex
BN21 1AA
Tel: 01323 412723

Glossary

Alopecia: Disease in which the hair falls out. Alopecia is a range of disorders in which some or all of the hair from the head and the body falls out. For details of types of alopecia, see Chapter 1.

Anagen phase: The phase of the hair cycle where the hair is growing. This is the longest phase of the cycle, and can last anything from two to ten years.

Antigens: These act as markers for immune cells. They are usually proteins. They are foreign to the body, and so when introduced stimulate an immune response, activating lymphocytes, the body's infection-fighting white blood cells. The surface of antigens has regions that bind to receptor molecules on the surface of lymphocytes. This stimulates the lymphocytes to multiply and initiate the immune response.

Attachment theory: A theory put forward by psychologists suggesting that our behaviour, our responses to the environment (including getting alopecia), depends to at least some extent on how successfully we attach to or bond with people, beginning with our parents at an early age. Our attachment patterns are said to be fairly stable throughout life.

Autoimmune disease: A disorder resulting from problems with the immune system.

Behaviourism: A perspective in psychology particularly popular during the first half of the twentieth century, and still popularly used for the effective treatment of a range of psychological disorders.

Catagen phase: The phase of the hair cycle where the hair follicle is resting.

Catecholamine: Common stress hormone. Naturally occurring amines that function as neurotransmitters and hormones within the body.

Chemotherapy: A set of chemical treatments used mainly for counteracting cancer. One of the main side-effects can be alopecia.

Clinical psychologist: A psychologist specially trained to deal with psychological disorders. Clinical psychologists typically employ a range of treatment strategies to help people resolve their problems.

Coping: The ability to deal with stress. 'Coping' is a very general term used to describe the different ways we deal with our problems. We might use emotion-focused coping, where we depend on our emotions to help us through a problem; or we might use cognitive processing, where we logically think through a problem; or we might use denial, where we refuse to acknowledge that there is a problem!

Corticosteroids: Major stress hormones. Corticosteroids are commonly used to treat alopecia.

Counsellor: Someone who is trained to listen to people's problems and help resolve them. There are many different types of counsellors, working from different perspectives. Some are better trained than others.

Cytokines: Any of a group of proteins that are released by one cell to regulate the function of another cell, thus serving as intercellular chemical messengers. Cytokines effect changes in cellular behaviour which are important in a number of physiological processes, including reproduction, growth and development, and injury repair, and they have a role in the immune system's defence against disease-causing organisms.

Dermatitis: A range of skin disorders. Dermatitis (or eczema) is inflammation of the skin and is usually characterized by redness, swelling, blister formation, and oozing and itching.

Dermatology: The study of skin and skin disorders. Dermatologists are specialist doctors responsible for a range of skin complaints, including alopecia.

Follicle: The hair cell.

Genes: These are units of hereditary information that occupy a fixed position on a chromosome. Genes direct the synthesis of proteins in order to have their effect. We all have many thousands of genes on our chromosomes; they are responsible for many of our physical and psychological characteristics. Researchers are only just starting to understand the details of how particular genes work.

Glucocorticoids: These are related to the stress response and help to suppress the immune system and act as anti-inflammatories.

Homeostasis: The process by which the body maintains balance. Homeostasis is any self-regulating process by which a biological system will try to maintain stability while adjusting to conditions that are optimal for survival.

Immune system: One of the main protective systems for ensuring health. The immune system is a complex set of defence mechanisms which protect us from a range of environmental problems.

Inflammatory response: This is the most primitive of bodily protective mechanisms. Damaged tissue may become infected, which triggers the inflammatory response.

Keratin: This is the fibrous structural protein of hair, nails, horn, hoofs, wool and feathers, and of the epithelial cells in the outermost layers of the skin.

Lymph nodes: Crucial part of the immune system. It is here that the white blood cells are generated.

Male-pattern baldness: Also known as alopecia androgenetica. This is what we know as the ordinary baldness experienced mainly by men as they age. In a minority of cases, women also experience male-pattern baldness, particularly after the menopause.

Minoxidil: One of the most common topical corticosteroids used to treat alopecia.

Neuropeptides: A wide range of hormones which regulate many aspects of behaviour.

Post-traumatic stress disorder (PTSD): A psychological disorder resulting from a person experiencing a traumatic event such as death, injury, disaster, rape or war. It is characterized by intrusive re-experiencing, avoidance, emotional numbing and hyperarousal. People with PTSD may also experience disorders such as depression or substance abuse.

Psychiatrist: A medical practitioner who has received psychological training.

Psychoneuroimmunology: The study of the relationship between behaviour, the nervous system and the immune system. Many physical disorders can have psychological causes mediated by a dysfunctioning immune system.

Stress: This refers to any strain that disturbs the functioning of the person. We respond to stress using a range of defences, and if these defences are overpowered, it may result in a psychological or psychosomatic disorder. 'Stress' is an overused word that refers to a) actual damage to a system, b) the perceived damage to the system, or c) the thing in the environment that causes the damage to the system.

Substance P: This acts as a neurotransmitter in the central nervous system. It is related to stress.

Telogen phase: The phase of the hair cycle where the hair is being shed. This lasts between one and three months. The hair must be shed in order to prepare for the next growth (anagen) phase.

Trichotillomania: An obsessive-compulsive disorder characterized by pulling out one's hair.

Index